The Liver Remedy

Natural Liver Health Solutions to Address Cirrhosis, Inflammation, Fatty Liver, Hepatitis, NAFLD and NASH, Hepatic Disorders

Dr. Steven Scott

Copyright @2024

The content in this book is for general informational purposes only and is not meant to be medical advice. Its objective is to support and educate readers who are interested in learning more about liver diseases and how to manage them.

Disclaimer: The information presented in this book is not specific medical advice for any individual and should not substitute medical advice from a health professional. If you have (or think you may have) a medical problem, speak to your doctor or a health professional immediately about your risk and possible treatments. Do not engage in any care or treatment without consulting a medical professional.

Table of Contents

CHAPTER 1

Your Extraordinary Liver

Whenever the liver is brought up, a viral infection like hepatitis B or C is typically brought up. Because of this, the majority of people have very little knowledge about their liver and its true importance. We would expire very soon without a liver. Although the full scope of this connection is yet unknown to us, we do know that when one organ, like the liver, malfunctions, other organs will also change in function. Strangely, the brain is included in this as well. And they do exchange messages with one another. We must never forget that all of our tissues and organs are in continual communication with one another, and that the failure of one organ has a detrimental effect on several other tissues and organs. Assuming organs can or do function in isolation is one common error individuals make. These are frequent queries: What functions do the pancreas and liver perform?

The liver, which is the largest organ in the body, is reddish-brown in color and weighs 1500 grams, or around three pounds. Tucked under the ribs on the right side of our bodies, it resembles a wedge. On the right side, it is partially attached to the diaphragm's bottom. The liver is important enough to be positioned beneath the rib cage to protect it from harm. The liver's lower margin typically stops short of the lowest rib. As you may remember, your doctor will begin pressing on your abdomen on the right side, just below the ribs, when performing a physical examination. This helps them determine the approximate location of the liver's margins. Your liver's lower margin will be below the rightmost rib if it is enlarged. The doctor is more concerned if the liver protrudes farther down since this could mean that your liver is larger and may even be damaged or malfunctioning. Your liver is unique in another way as well because, in addition to receiving blood normally from an artery and a vein, it also receives blood specifically from the intestines. The hepatic portal vein system is the name given to this unique group of veins. It's interesting to note that 75% of the blood fed to the liver comes from this particular portal vein. The hepatic portal vein transports various substances to the liver, including endocrine secretions from the pancreas, special endocrine secretions from the gastrointestinal tract, red blood cells, and breakdown products of blood cells (old blood cells are eliminated by the spleen), as well as nutrients and toxic materials from the intestines. The oxygenation of the blood in the hepatic portal vein is extremely low. Compared to most other organs, the liver can function with less oxygen. The liver's drainage system is quite intricate, involving both unique sinusoidal capillaries and the common hepatic veins. Because of this configuration, every liver cell has direct access to the blood supply, which is necessary for the liver to carry out all of its complex processes. The lymphatic system provides an extra drainage system. Its numerous blood arteries contribute to the liver's high vascularity. There is a very real risk of fatal bleeding from liver injuries.

Microscopic View of Your Liver

In order to produce and/or store all the proteins, carbs, lipids, hormones, various vitamins, iron, and other elements your body requires for optimal health specially to shield you from harmful substances within your body your liver functions like a vast factory.

If you were to look at your liver under a microscope, you would see that it is made up of many lobules, which are small lobes with six sides (hexagrams). Within these subdivisions are blood vessels, canals (also known as ducts), and sinusoids. Hepatocytes, the cells that make up the majority of the mass of the liver, are scattered throughout these vascular spaces. Although these cells play a major role in the liver's functions, other cells have specific roles that are as important. These lobules are made to enable the surface of the liver cells to be exposed to the bloodstream to a great extent. This allows the liver cells to take up nutrients, toxins, and hormones from the bloodstream and release all the different products that the liver cells produce back into the bloodstream.

The liver doesn't take a break. The liver is always active because it is your body's first line of defense against harmful substances entering your body and even producing them. It also plays a crucial role in providing all the nutrients, proteins, and structural elements needed for all the cells in your body. It's important for you to learn more about how your liver influences all of your body's organs, including your brain. Why? Because of this, even at low concentrations, your brain is very susceptible to harmful compounds in the bloodstream. The function of other organs, including the heart, kidneys, lungs, pancreas, and brain, gradually declines when the liver fails.

Functions of the Liver

One of the body's most important organs, the liver carries out a variety of tasks that are essential to general health and wellbeing. The following are a few of the main functions of the liver:

- Nutrient metabolism (Proteins, Carbohydrates, Lipids (Fats) Vitamins/minerals).
- Detoxification (Pharmaceutical drugs, Illicit drugs, Food toxins, Toxins produced during metabolism or by illness, Toxins produced by bacteria in the GI tract)
- Nutrient Storage
- Immunity
- Blood coagulation
- Cholesterol metabolism
- Bile production
- Endocrine-like functions

Nutrient metabolism

The liver plays a critical role in food metabolism, turning proteins, lipids, and carbs into energy the body needs. It breaks down meals into carbs, lipids, and proteins while processing blood from the small intestine. These are the duties carried out by hepatocytes, which comprise 65% of the liver cells. Additionally, the liver contributes to the breakdown and absorption of fat by creating bile, which facilitates the absorption of fat-soluble vitamins. Due to significant amounts of undigested fat, liver illness patients may have white stool, and liver disorders patients may have shortages in fat-soluble vitamins. Moreover, the liver takes up blood glucose and stores it as glycogen. The liver releases some glucose back into the bloodstream by breaking down glycogen if blood sugar levels drop too low. The majority of the body's circulating proteins, such as albumin, lipoproteins, and glycoproteins involved in the transport of cholesterol, are produced by the liver. Because liver diseases deplete albumin, they can cause edema in the limbs. The liver also produces cholesterol.

Detoxification

The liver is the primary organ involved in detoxification, and the cells most exposed to the blood passing through the liver are called hepatocytes. Phase I and Phase II metabolic systems facilitate liver detoxification. The first line of defense against pharmaceutical medicines, steroids, hormones, and xenobiotics is phase I detoxification. The most crucial stage of detoxification is phase II, which changes substances that are insoluble in water into substances that are soluble in water and may be eliminated by the kidneys through the gastrointestinal tract and urine.

The body produces a great deal of internal poisons in addition to environmental poisoning. Every day, more than three pounds of cells perish, making place for fresh, healthy ones.

In the last 30 days, about half of all Americans have taken at least one prescription medication, and it doesn't even account for the enormous volume of OTC medications that people consume. Your liver's functions are the reason these medications even function in our bodies. These medications are processed by your liver; nevertheless, even while our livers' metabolism of these substances produces their intended benefits, these modified compounds may also be harmful. It's true that this requires careful balancing. The majority of medications you take, whether they are prescribed or over-the-counter, need to be digested in order to function. The enzymes in your liver can accomplish this by changing them into a form that your body can use more efficiently or by making them less toxic so that they can be safely eliminated. Since they account for 70–80% of the enzymes involved in drug metabolism, the metabolic enzymes produced by the cytochrome P450 (CYP450) gene group (Phase I) are the most significant of all.

The detoxification process of the liver itself increases the toxicity of certain medicines. Stated differently, the medicine becomes significantly more toxic due to the liver than it would have otherwise. The enzymes in your liver can accomplish this by changing them into a form that your body can use more efficiently or by making them less toxic so that they can be safely eliminated. Since they account for 70–80% of the enzymes involved in drug metabolism, the metabolic enzymes produced by the cytochrome P450 (CYP450) gene group (Phase I) are the most significant of all.

The detoxification process of the liver itself increases the toxicity of certain medicines. Stated differently, the medicine becomes significantly more toxic due to the liver than it would have otherwise. Acetaminophen (Tylenol) is a prime example of a drug that the liver's Phase I detoxification mechanism greatly increases in toxicity. One of the more dangerous medications on the market, acetaminophen is the reason why a large number of patients require liver transplants. With over 100,000 calls annually, this medication is the main reason for calls to the Poison Control Center and is also the primary cause of 56,000 ER visits.

Storage

As we saw with glycogen and fatty acids, your liver also stores vitamins A, D, E, and K, which your body can use as needed. Your body may survive on these stored nutrients for a considerable amount of time thanks to the protective action of your liver during periods of nutrient scarcity and hunger. Furthermore, vitamins and minerals required for metabolism as well as tissue and cell repair are also stored in your liver.

Immunity

An essential component of the immune system is the liver. The linings of the lungs and GI tract are the two primary points of contact between the inside and outside of the body. Bacteria, viruses, and fungi can enter the lower gastrointestinal tract by food and contaminated objects that we place in our mouths. Immune cells are concentrated most heavily in the GI tract walls and respiratory system tubes (lungs, trachea, and nasal cavity). In the event that these microbes manage to bypass the intestines' first line of defense, the hepatic portal circulation system transports them straight to the liver. The body's largest concentration of phagocytic immune cells, which devour these microbes like a ravenous shark, are found in the liver. Like other parts of the body, the liver can launch a standard immunological reaction if things go worse.

It is well known that the immune system's capacity to eradicate invasive microbes declines with age. Paradoxically, an aging body might experience a significant rise in inflammation due to immune system dysfunction. When there is inadequate immune activity, there may be high levels of inflammation. You'll see that immune system function is completely dependent on proper diet. This includes getting enough fat, protein, and carbohydrates as well as all the vitamins and minerals, particularly:

- Vitamin C
- Natural vitamin E (mixed tocopherols and tocotrienols)
- B-complex vitamins
- Carotenoids
- Magnesium
- Zinc
- Selenium
- Manganese
- Magnesium
- Copper

The discovery that even a single deficit, such as pyridoxine (B6), thiamine (B1), or riboflavin (B2), can significantly impair immune function is particularly significant. There is proof that certain vital nutrients can weaken immunity even at low-to-normal levels (subclinical deficits). These crucial, potentially life-saving discoveries are rarely discussed in the medical community. This implies that dietary supplements have the potential to determine whether a person has a healthy life, bad health, or, frequently, passes away. The body needs to create trillions of white blood cells—lymphocytes, neutrophils, macrophages, and monocytes—during an infection in order to combat the invasive microbes.

Keeping Your Brain Sharp and Safe

Toxin accumulation in the bloodstream is the main thing the liver does. These poisons have the potential to impair brain function in cases of severe liver disease, which can alter behavior, mood, and sleep patterns. These modifications may come either quickly or gradually over time. Depression, anxiety, and difficulty focusing are examples of mild symptoms. As the condition worsens, patients may have tremors in the hands, spasms in the muscles, loss of balance, disorientation, and difficulties focusing. We refer to these symptoms as "brain fog." People who suffer from other illnesses including frailty or chronic inflammatory disorders may also experience brain fog. Thus, keeping the liver healthy may assist people with various conditions remain cognitively intact.

CHAPTER 2

Liver Protects and Maintains Health

To various people, detoxification might signify different things. Detoxification is loosely defined as eating a healthy diet. Actually, this is not just the body's first line of defense against poisonous elements found in food; it can also activate the body's detoxification processes within its numerous tissues and cells, clearing the body of these dangerous substances.

Every cell has detoxification systems of some kind, such as unique compounds like glutathione, which can bind and eliminate various harmful metals including lead, mercury, and cadmium in addition to acting as a potent antioxidant. Another chemical that aids in cellular detoxification is called metallothionein, which gets rid of dangerous metals like arsenic, cadmium, mercury, and lead. The gastrointestinal tract's (GI tract) lining cells and the kidneys are two other important detoxification systems. Because they serve as the body's first line of defense against harmful substances that can enter through eating and drinking, the cells lining the gastrointestinal system are particularly significant. The liver continues to be the body's primary detoxifying organ. It purges the body's circulation of harmful compounds that are absorbed through the skin or breathed into the lungs in addition to entering through the GI tract.

Let's examine in more detail how the liver rids itself of these dangerous substances now. To deal with these dangerous substances, the liver employs a two-tier system known as phase I and phase II detoxification.

Phase I Detoxification

Many detoxifying enzymes categorized as CYP-450 enzymes (also simply referred to as P-450 enzymes) are utilized by the liver. Chemicals are toxic due to specific, sometimes extremely precise, structural features of their molecules. The liver will chemically change these harmful substances to make them less toxic so they are safe. The first line of defense is the phase I enzymes, although it is not flawless.

The CYP-450 enzymes in the liver often try to detoxify a harmful molecule by attaching specific chemical groups to it in order to lessen its toxicity. These involve giving the hazardous molecule chemical groups such as hydroxyl, carboxyl, and amino groups attached.

Pharmaceutical companies made adjustments for whatever modifications the liver would make to their products because they knew their products would be processed by the liver's chemical factory. Most significantly, they estimated the amount of time needed for the medication to be neutralized and eliminated by the liver enzymes. For instance, the doctor would have to recommend giving the medication every six hours in order for it to be effective if it took the liver six hours to metabolize and eliminate it. According to studies, several CYP enzyme types are in charge of eliminating or detoxifying particular substances.

Numerous procarcinogen molecules, or substances that need to undergo a chemical conversion in order to cause cancer, are found in nature. They are frequently transformed by the liver's phase I detoxification mechanism into substances that cause cancer. This is observed with several pesticides, herbicides, and fungicides, as well as with naturally occurring carcinogens like aflatoxin. These procarcinogens are being transformed by your liver into potent carcinogens. For instance, polycyclic aromatic hydrocarbons (PAH), heterocyclic aromatic amines, and polychlorinated biphenyls (PCBs) can all be transformed into completely hazardous substances by the detoxifying enzyme CYP1.

Phase I detoxification, as we have seen, is generally quite effective; yet, on sometimes, mistakes are made, and the situation worsens or even becomes fatal. Acetaminophen, or Tylenol, is a prime example of how phase I detoxification can seriously harm or even completely kill the liver and kidneys due to this medication. The liver has a strong fallback mechanism for situations like this. The phase II system, which functions in concert with phase I but through a distinct set of mechanisms, is this backup system.

Phase II Detoxification

We discovered that phase I detoxification works by adding molecules that lower toxicity, which in turn reduces the majority of the toxicity of harmful compounds circulating in human blood. Unfortunately, this also rendered the hazardous substances insoluble in water, which may be dangerous as they remain in the liver and can do a great deal of harm there.

Phase II detoxification chemically alters these harmful compounds to make them water soluble in order to stop this. By doing this, the harmful substances can be removed from the body by the gastrointestinal tract through bile and the kidneys through urine. We refer to step II detoxification as conjugation in chemical terms. This refers to a chemical procedure in which the poisonous substance is made water soluble by adding specific compounds to it. This procedure is carried out by certain enzymes that are soluble in water. Among them are:

- Glucuronic acid (glucuronyl transferases)
- Sulfate (sulfotransferases)
- Glutathione (glutathione transferases)
- Amino acids (amino acid transferases)
- Acetyl groups (N-acetyl transferases)
- Methyl groups (N-and O-methyltransferases)

When confronted with internal hazardous compounds or large toxic loads like junk food or agrichemicals, the liver's detoxifying enzymes are elevated. Hormone metabolism may be impacted by abnormal liver function, raising the possibility of hormone-dependent malignancies. Additionally, these enzymes alter with age, pregnancy, and pollution. Deficits in glucuronyl transferase enzymes can raise the risk of neurological illnesses such as Parkinson's disease and colon cancer. Research emphasize how crucial detoxifying enzymes are to preserving general health.

Glutathione-S-transferase is used in phase II detoxification, and acetaminophen depletes this enzyme. Detoxifying medications that include aromatic amines or hydrazine requires the activity of this enzyme. Methionine, vitamins B12, B6, folate, and betaine are examples of natural substances that supply methyl groups for the metabolism of estrogen and detoxification. Another crucial methyl donor is SAMe.

Foods, Plant Extracts, and Additional Nutritious Supplements Impacting the Detoxification Process

The liver's detoxification process can be modified by plants and plant extracts; however, the dose is important. For instance, the phase I enzyme CYP1A1 can be stimulated by curcumin, an extract from turmeric, but at greater doses, it can be suppressed. This may stop the production of chemicals that cause cancer. Nevertheless, if a pharmaceutical medication needs this enzyme for metabolism, inhibiting the detoxifying enzyme may have negative effects. Although resveratrol and cauliflowers can activate this enzyme, their anticancer properties can mitigate its effects. Elevated concentrations of these plants may impact phase I detoxification; nonetheless, it's crucial to take these interactions into account, particularly in relation to pharmaceutical medications.

Phase II function is also influenced by plants; cruciferous vegetables increase UDP-glucuronosyltransferase activity. These enzymes are also stimulated by meals high in magnesium, such as halibut, almonds, cashews, spinach, oats, peanuts, and wheat bran. Due to its ability to eliminate harmful compounds from the body, the phase II system is the most crucial for detoxification protection.

Glutathione levels in the liver and other cells are raised by natural items such as curcumin, silymarin, folic acid, NAC, duck, egg yolks, cheese, red peppers, garlic, onions, and R-lipoic acid. Glutathione functions as glutathione-S-transferase and is a potent detoxifying agent. Certain foods raise the level of sulfur to aid in detoxifying. Certain natural chemicals regulate detoxification enzymes, increasing their activity when they're lacking or decreasing it when it's too high. These substances' anti-inflammatory, anti-carcinogenic, antibacterial, antioxidant, and regeneration-promoting qualities help shield the liver.

Particular Liver Guards

Considering its significance, liver health maintenance is essential. Supplements are a common way that specific liver protectors can help shield the liver from harm and promote liver function. When it comes to supporting general well-being or improving liver function as a result of exposure to pollutants or lifestyle factors, these supplements can be very helpful.

Curcumin

Turmeric extract, or curcumin, has many health advantages, such as preventing cancer, treating mental diseases, preventing cytokine storms, reducing autoimmune symptoms, and protecting the liver. It contains anti-inflammatory and antioxidant qualities, safeguards glutathione, replenishes liver enzymes, prevents lipid peroxidation, and promotes liver regeneration. But since curcumin absorbs poorly when taken alone, it's best to take it alongside vitamin C half an hour before meals.

Turmeric extract, or curcumin, has many health advantages, such as preventing cancer, treating mental diseases, preventing cytokine storms, reducing autoimmune symptoms, and protecting the liver. It contains anti-inflammatory and antioxidant qualities, safeguards glutathione, replenishes liver enzymes, prevents lipid peroxidation, and promotes liver regeneration. But since curcumin absorbs poorly when taken alone, it's best to take it alongside vitamin C half an hour before meals.

Anthocyanins

Through antioxidant actions, enzyme suppression, and improved liver enzymes, the substance present in red wine, grapes, blueberries, blackberries, black currents, and red cabbage can protect the liver from chemical harm.

Apigenin

Flavonoids called apigenin, which are present in celery, oranges, onions, parsley, and grapefruit, have been demonstrated to shield mice against acetaminophen toxicity, promote liver tissue regeneration, lower lipid peroxidation, and raise glutathione levels.

Berberine

An ingredient found in Berberis aristate called berberine inhibits CYP-450 enzymes, which lowers the amount of procarcinogen chemicals that are transformed into carcinogenic compounds. Additionally, it treats insulin resistance, lessens inflammation and fatty liver issues, and may even aid with type 2 diabetes.

Hesperidin

This particular flavonoid can be found in citrus fruits like grapefruits, tangerines, and oranges. Numerous investigations have demonstrated that this flavonoid shields the liver by restoring antioxidant enzymes, lowering inflammation, and preventing the loss of liver cells. Hesperidin is available as a supplement and has a great safety record.

Luteolin

Many fruits and vegetables contain this flavonoid, but it is particularly abundant in sweet green peppers, green hot chili peppers, celery, pumpkins, and artichokes. Strong anti-inflammatory and antioxidant properties of luteolin have been demonstrated, as well as the ability to replenish and restore liver enzymes. It also repairs damaged liver tissue and keeps the liver's supply of glutathione from running low. It also has the added benefit of lowering brain fog.

Meso-Zeaxanthin

One carotenoid that is essential for shielding the eye's macula is meso-zeaxanthin. Furthermore, it has demonstrated remarkable efficacy in hepatoprotection through the elevation of glutathione levels, the restoration of liver enzymes, the action of a potent antioxidant, and the repair of liver cell damage resulting from exposure to harmful chemicals like acetaminophen. It is available for purchase as an add-on.

Pterostilbene

Blueberries have a high concentration of this chemical. It is transformed into resveratrol after leaving the GI tract. It provides a higher degree of safety and is much more readily absorbed than resveratrol. Research has demonstrated that this substance is a potent antioxidant, strong anti-inflammatory, shields the liver from acetaminophen toxicity, lowers lipid peroxidation, boosts liver antioxidant enzymes, blocks inflammatory cytokines, and heals damaged liver cells. It is available for purchase as an add-on.

Schisandra

This plant's compounds have demonstrated potent liver-protective properties. Schisandra yields several separate chemicals, all of which have been shown to protect the liver. The plant's antioxidant properties, suppression of lipid peroxidation, restoration of the liver's enzymes, decrease in some CYP-450 enzymes, enhanced activation of the primary antioxidant system (Nrf2) in the liver cells, and stimulation of liver cell repair all contribute to protection. This substance has a favorable safety profile and is available for purchase as a supplement.

Silybin (Silymarin)

The majority of people are aware of silymarin and believe it to be the primary natural substance that protects the liver. It may not be as effective as some of the other substances mentioned before, despite the fact that it possesses outstanding liver protecting characteristics. It has been demonstrated to considerably lessen acetaminophen toxicity, stop glutathione depletion, and decrease lipid peroxidation. It is helpful for many other medical conditions and has an excellent safety record. It is particularly beneficial for treating and preventing different types of cancer, enhancing prostate health, and safeguarding brain function.

Zinc

Controlling zinc intake is important to prevent neurological impairment and is essential for good health. It increases the synthesis of metallothionein, a substance that is abundant in the liver and gastrointestinal system. It is necessary for metabolic processes and possesses antioxidant qualities as well. Overconsumption of zinc can result in copper deficiency, which can induce sideroblastic anemia, headaches, and excessive perspiration. Take a zinc supplement every other day, no more than 15 mg daily, to avoid this. Because copper is harmful at greater dosages, it should only be consumed in moderation. Because their livers already contain large amounts of copper, cirrhosis patients should refrain from taking copper supplements or eating foods high in copper.

Magnesium

Magnesium shortage is universal in cirrhosis and particularly common in liver disorders. Even worse, as in the case of cirrhosis, a magnesium deficit can exacerbate and hasten liver deterioration. A magnesium deficit will exacerbate inflammation in the liver's tissues and reduce the mitochondria's capacity to synthesis energy, which exacerbates the processes that lead to liver damage—free radical production and lipid peroxidation.

Unfortunately, due to a decrease in the consumption of foods high in magnesium, such as leafy green vegetables, nuts, pumpkin seeds, spinach, and tuna, magnesium shortage is rather widespread in the modern world. High alcohol intake significantly reduces magnesium levels, as does stress and inflammation, particularly long-term inflammation. According to studies, supplementing with magnesium and selenium (as selenomethionine) enhances the liver's defense against lipid peroxidation and free radical damage.

CHAPTER 3

Liver Tests and Symptoms

This book intends to help readers maintain a healthy liver by outlining the numerous risks it faces from outside sources, chemicals consumed—knowingly or unknowingly—and incurable illnesses. It talks about several liver disorders, some of which have particular symptoms and diagnostic tests, and others of which have common symptoms and diagnostic tests. The chapter goes into great length on these subjects, emphasizing the significance of liver health and the different functions it serves in the body.

Signs and Symptoms of Liver Disease

Due of its advanced stage, liver disease is frequently disregarded, resulting in severe damage to the liver. The disease doesn't show symptoms until it's advanced because too much good tissue is lost despite the liver's capacity to regenerate. Gastroenterologist Dr. Anrug Maheshwari of Mercy Medical Center's Institute for Digestive Health and

Liver Disease highlights the need of managing liver disease prophylactically. When liver disease is advanced, jaundice may be the initial symptom, but most other symptoms also show up. In order to avoid complications such as serious liver damage and scarring, early identification is essential.

This is a major reason to make sure your doctor is paying attention to you if you suspect you may have a liver illness.

Symptoms of Liver Disease

Jaundice

Jaundice is the medical term for yellowing of the skin and eyes. When your body produces too much bilirubin, jaundice develops. In the liver, the breakdown of dead red blood cells produces bilirubin, a yellow pigment. Old red blood cells and bilirubin are normally eliminated by the liver. Jaundice may be the first symptom to manifest in most liver disorders because most of them don't have any early warning signs. If this occurs to you, be sure to see your doctor very once. A blockage of the liver drainage system, such as the bile ducts or intrahepatic channels, is typically indicated by jaundice.

Pain

 a dull ache somewhat below the ribs in the right side of the abdomen. This may be a sign of liver pain, which can have several causes, such as liver cancer, cirrhosis, hepatitis, ascites (fluid in the abdomen), liver failure, or an abscess in the liver. Due to its proximity to the liver, gas trapped in the right hepatic flexure of the colon can produce a similar kind of pain, particularly in those with irritable colon disease.

Weight Loss

Loss of appetite or unexplained weight loss may indicate severe liver disease. Swelling and Pain in the Abdomen An imbalance of proteins and other chemicals caused by a malfunctioning liver can lead to ascites, a disorder that can be indicated by a bloated abdomen. It also happens when the hepatic veins are obstructed. This could be the result of advanced cirrhosis.

Swelling

Leg and ankle swelling, which frequently coexists with ascites, might also be an indicator of more severe liver disease brought on by cirrhosis. Itchy Skin Bile salt buildup beneath the skin may be a symptom of liver illness and cause excruciating itching.

Dark Urine

The kidneys' excretion of bilirubin might cause urine to become black. Excessive bilirubin levels can be caused by bile duct blockage, inflammation, or other abnormalities of the liver cells. The breakdown of red blood cells in the liver produces bilirubin, an orange-yellow pigment. Bile is used to expel it.

Oddly Colored Stool

Bloody or tarry stools, or pale stools: Pale stools may be a sign of an issue with the liver or another component of the biliary drainage system. Light-colored or extremely pale stool that floats suggest a bile deficit that prevents the absorption of fat. This may be the result of other liver issues or occlusion of the bile duct. Blood traveling through the gastrointestinal system is the cause of black, tarry stools, which can occur in severe liver disease. This can suggest an urgent medical situation.

Prolonged Fatigue

Although the exact origin of extreme fatigue, exhaustion, and tiredness is unknown, it is an indication of advanced liver disease. Certain doctors speculate that low energy levels could be caused by a build-up of pollutants or altered hormone levels; still others think it is because of alterations in brain chemistry brought on by reduced liver function.

Nausea or Vomiting

This is an additional indication of severe liver illness since it prevents the body from processing and getting rid of toxins. Another indicator of advanced liver disease is the propensity to bruise easily, as this suggests that the liver is no longer able to create the necessary proteins for blood to clot and is no longer working normally.

The Liver Disease Stages

Liver illness comes in various forms, each distinct from the other yet sharing some characteristics. One of these is that a lot of liver disorders, though not all of them, have distinct phases that the organ goes through as it gets more and more damaged. The fundamental risk is the same regardless of the type of liver illness you have—whether it was caused by a virus, drugs, immunological disease, alcohol, or another condition. The liver will sustain so much damage that it is unable to operate normally. An illustration of the phases the liver might go through is given below. As you'll see, the liver can regain function and halt the decline if this disease process is interrupted early on.

The Healthy Liver

A healthy liver is free from disease and able to carry out all of its vital tasks, such as breaking down meals, storing glycogen for energy, storing fat-soluble vitamins, and shielding the body from toxins. In addition, it has the ability to replenish itself, so even harm can cause it to grow back.

Inflammation

An inflammatory response in the liver is the first indication of the condition. This indicates that it has been hurt and is attempting to mend. This is what happens when you cut your finger; the injured region gets painful and red. It is clear that it has grown inflamed. The issue with liver inflammation is that it's frequently a low-grade, smoldering, chronic inflammation. This means that the inflammation is hidden deep within the body, and if it isn't stopped, the damage to the liver will continue to grow.

Fibrosis

The irritated liver starts to scar if the inflammation is not treated. This indicates a process called fibrosis, in which healthy liver tissue is replaced by scarred tissue. The duties that healthy liver tissue can perform cannot be performed by scarred tissue. Even worse, damaged tissue can accumulate and impede hepatic channels and blood flow within the liver, further damaging the organ.

Cirrhosis

When soft, healthy liver tissue is replaced with hard, damaged tissue, the condition is known as cirrhosis. The quantity of healthy liver tissue decreases as cirrhosis worsens, and the liver will finally fail if treatment is not received. Liver cancer can also result from cirrhosis. Following a diagnosis of cirrhosis, the goal of treatment is to preserve the remaining viable liver tissue while attempting to limit the progression of the disease.

End-Stage Liver Disease

This contains a subset of cirrhosis patients who have untreatable symptoms, many of which were previously mentioned. Another name for this stage could be liver failure. Right now, the only available treatment is a liver transplant.

Liver Disease Diagnostic Tests

Tests are performed to evaluate liver function and find any underlying abnormalities in order to diagnose liver disease. Effective management and therapy may depend on early discovery, which these diagnostic tests can provide. A few typical diagnostic procedures used to assess liver health are as follows:

Blood Tests

Liver Function Tests (LFTs)

The liver function panel, also known as the hepatic function panel, is made up of multiple tests because there isn't just one particular test that is used to determine how well the liver is performing. This test measures the amounts of albumin, bilirubin, total protein, and liver enzymes in your blood using certain values. Excessive or insufficient levels might point to illness or damage to the liver. This panel is included in the lab tests that are administered during a general physical, which is advantageous because it can be used to screen for liver issues in otherwise healthy individuals.

The following are typical causes of increased liver enzymes:

- Over-the-counter drugs, particularly pain medications such as acetaminophen (Tylenol, etc.)
- Certain prescription medications, including cholesterol-lowering statin drugs
- Drinking alcohol

- Hepatitis A, B, and C
- Nonalcoholic fatty liver disease
- Obesity

Less common causes include the following:

- Alcoholic hepatitis (liver inflammation caused by alcohol)
- Autoimmune hepatitis (liver inflammation caused by an autoimmune disease such as celiac disease, rheumatoid arthritis, or hyperthyroidism (Grave's disease or Hashimoto's thyroiditis)
- Cytomegalovirus (a common virus that may cause no problems except in women who are pregnant or people with weakened immune systems) • Epstein–Barr virus
- Hemochromatosis (too much iron stored in the body)
- Liver cancer
- Mononucleosis
- Polymyositis (an uncommon inflammatory disease that causes weakness)
- Sepsis
- Thyroid disorders

- Wilson's disease (too much copper stored in the body)

Liver Tests Often Disregarded

Although the liver function test is useful, physicians frequently ignore it. It's critical to preserve lab testing and inquire about unusual findings. If results seem strange, run the test again to be sure everything is normal. These tests' progressive rise suggests a serious illness. It's frequently advised in a variety of circumstances.

- To monitor side effects if you're taking a medication that is known to affect the liver
- To check for damage from liver infections, such as hepatitis B and hepatitis C
- To check for a reason for the symptoms
- To monitor people at risk for liver problems if, for instance, they have high triglycerides, diabetes, high blood pressure, or have gallbladder disease or anemia
- To monitor heavy alcohol drinkers

What a Liver Function Test Measures

A Liver Function Test (LFT), sometimes referred to as a hepatic panel, assesses a number of blood components, including proteins, enzymes, and other chemicals, that are connected to the health and function of the liver. These examinations can detect the existence of liver damage or illness and aid in tracking the course of a condition or the efficacy of treatment. The main elements assessed in a liver function test are as follows, along with their respective meanings:

Protein

Made up of molecules known as amino acids, protein is a vital component required for fluid balance, energy production, tissue maintenance and repair, and immune system support. Your blood's protein level will be monitored by your doctor to ensure that it supports the liver's functioning.

Albumin

A particular protein called albumin is made in the liver and is vital for healing as well as carrying drugs and other materials through the blood and assisting in the prevention of blood spilling out of blood vessels.

Bilirubin

When hemoglobin, the protein found in red blood cells, and aged red blood cells degrade, a chemical known as bilirubin is created. Bilirubin levels in the blood should normally be extremely low. A jaundiced color, which is symptomatic of liver disease, may result from an excessive elevation. Ammonia might accumulate if the liver is not working correctly. The brain gets poisoned by ammonia.

Enzymes

The body produces enzymes to expedite chemical reactions, including blood coagulation, digestion, detoxification, and energy metabolism. Certain liver issues can be diagnosed with the aid of abnormal enzyme levels. Among them are: Alkali-Surfactant The enzyme alkaline phosphatase, or ALP, is measured in this test. The intestines and kidneys also produce some ALP, but the liver and bone are the primary locations for production. An excessively high level may be a sign of a blocked bile flow, vitamin D insufficiency, cancer that has migrated to the bone, damaged liver cells, or bone diseases such Paget's disease.

Aspartate Aminotransferase (AST)

Red blood cells, the liver, heart muscle tissue, the pancreas, and the kidneys are typically home to this enzyme. The amount is normally low; an excessively high level may be a sign of liver or cardiac disease.

Alanine Aminotransferase (ALT)

Another enzyme that is mostly present in the liver is called ALT; nevertheless, minor levels are also present in the kidneys, heart, muscles, and pancreas. This test has the potential to reveal liver disease as well.

Blood Clotting Tests

The coagulation process is carried out by the liver. The organ's ability to clot blood can be examined using two different techniques.

- **Partial thromboplastin time (PTT):** This test is done to check for blood clotting problems.

- **Prothrombin time (PT):** This test is frequently performed to find out if a patient is taking warfarin (Coumadin), a blood thinner, at the recommended dosage. It can also identify issues with blood coagulation.

Imaging Tests

- **Ultrasound**: This is a non-invasive test done to detect many liver conditions, including cancer, cirrhosis, or gallstones.
- **MRI scan (computed tomography):** More precise imaging of the liver and other abdominal organs can be obtained using an MRI scan. An MRI scan of the biliary system and liver, for example, can assess the presence of tumors, injuries, bleeding, infections, abscesses, blockages, or other disorders in the liver, gallbladder, or related organs. Due to the lack of radiation, an MRI is safer than a CT scan.

Liver Biopsy

During a liver biopsy, a needle is used to take a little sample of liver tissue. After that, a microscope is used to look at this sample in order to assess the level of liver illness or damage. Although intrusive, it offers conclusive details regarding the state of the liver.

- **Liver biopsy:** A tiny needle is injected into the liver during a liver biopsy procedure to remove a sample of tissue, which is subsequently examined. A liver biopsy is typically carried out in order to make a number of medical diagnoses. It can be used, for instance, to determine the reason for persistently high liver enzymes, unexplained skin yellowing, liver abnormalities seen with non-invasive procedures like CT scans or ultrasounds, or unexplained liver enlargement.
- **Liver and spleen scan:** This test takes images of your liver using a tiny quantity of radioactive substance known as a radionuclide. Your spleen and liver can be seen in pictures taken by a gamma camera, a specialized tool. The spleen and liver collaborate closely in the synthesis and elimination of blood cells. This test can identify nonmalignant cysts,

abscesses, hematomas (bruise-like injuries), cirrhosis, hepatitis, and liver cancer. It can also track the progression of liver illness or injury.

CHAPTER 4

The All-American Diet Destroys Liver Function

The Western diet, sometimes referred to as the conventional American diet, is bad for the colon and intestines, heart attacks, strokes, atherosclerosis, and neurological illnesses. It also damages the liver. It consists of potatoes, corn, breads, red meat, processed foods, margarine, sweets, dairy products, refined cereals, and fructose. These foods weaken immunity, increase insulin resistance, obesity, inflammation, and diabetes. Coronary heart disease, type 2 diabetes, insulin resistance, metabolic syndrome, energy failure, and neurodegenerative illnesses are all associated with chronic inflammation. Additionally, residues from herbicides and pesticides that are harmful to the liver and can cause cancer are present in the diet.

The following are the elements of the typical American diet that are linked to liver damage:

- Excessively fatty foods

- Starchy foods high on the glycemic index and of high glycemic load
- Sugars (especially fructose and sucrose)
- Food additives and dyes (MSG, hydrolyzed protein extract, etc.)
- Artificial sweeteners (aspartame, Splenda, stevia, etc.)
- Gluten
- Lectins
- Toxic metals (lead, mercury, aluminum, and cadmium)

Fats and Oils

A balanced diet must include fats, with saturated fats being the most detrimental. Reduced insulin resistance, type 2 diabetes, cholesterol, and fat reduction can all be achieved with a high-fat, low-carb diet. Cell membrane function, immune control, ion trafficking, inflammation, blood pressure regulation, and gene expression regulation all depend on fats. If taken in large enough quantities, they may even function like prescription medications. Saturated, polyunsaturated, and monounsaturated fats are the three types of fats. Although polyunsaturated fats, such as omega-6 and omega-3 fats, are necessary for optimal health, they can also cause organ and tissue damage, inflammation, and the growth of cancer. Compounds with anti-inflammatory and anticancer properties, such as oleic acid and resveratrol, are found in monounsaturated oils like olive oil. Generally speaking, saturated fats—like coconut oil—are less dangerous than polyunsaturated omega-6 oils.

Trans Fats

The food industry launched Crisco, a lard-like fat, and partially hydrogenated cooking oils around 1910, which resulted in a high percentage of trans fats. These trans fats cause severe health problems, such as atherosclerosis and liver damage. Since the 1970s, the United States has seen a 62% growth in the consumption of oils and fats, with vegetable oils consuming the most. The food industry has been slowly working to eliminate trans fats, but even products with the label "contains no trans fats" may still include unhealthy oils.

Polyunsaturated Oils

Vegetable oils high in omega-6 have been connected to liver tumor invasion, cancer development, and inflammation. NASH, liver fibrosis, liver cirrhosis, and primary liver cancer can result from high consumption. Excessive consumption of these oils may also result in oxidative stress, increased liver enzymes, diabetes, insulin resistance, and fatty liver. A big offender is margarine, which contains maize oil and can boil and oxidize. Canola, peanut, corn, soybean, safflower, sunflower, and other polyunsaturated fats are hazardous and quickly oxidize. Omega-6 oils are present in most processed meals, and oxidation of omega-3 oils is also common. DHA and EPA found in omega-3 oils have the ability to be transformed into potent anti-inflammatory substances.

Liver diseases and Fats

According to recent study, unless a diet contains significant amounts of fructose or sucrose, saturated fats do not produce liver damage, fibrosis, or cirrhosis. Instead, they can cause fatty liver disorders on their own. Over the last 30 years, the amount of high fructose consumed has doubled, which has accelerated the onset of fatty liver disease (NAFLD). According to an adolescent study, 15.2% of boys and 52% of girls who were overweight or obese developed fatty livers. Sugar and polyunsaturated omega-6 oils found in soft drinks, sauces, and dressings were the most commonly linked foods to non-alcoholic fatty liver disease (NAFLD). Inflammation is brought on by the buildup of visceral fat, and severe inflammation, liver fibrosis, and insulin resistance can be brought on by the combination of MSG and trans fatty acids.

Tips to Cut Down on Fat

- Use extra virgin olive oil that is organic to make your own salad dressings.
- Instead of using cream, use half-and-half, or stay away from milk entirely.
- Cut back on the cheese you eat.
- For cooking, use coconut or olive oil instead, and to stop the oil from oxidizing, add turmeric.

- Eat less red meat and more fish, chicken, and pork that are low in mercury.
- Steer clear of processed foods and purchase meats that have been reared organically.
- Meals can be baked, grilled, boiled, steamed, or casseroled rather than fried.
- Steer clear of fatty pastries.
- Steer clear of pizza and other high-fat Mexican and Italian foods.

Starchy Foods

Complex carbohydrates known as starches can be converted into simple sugars or stored as glycogen. They are present in potatoes, pasta, breads, rice, and grains. These carbs, which come in two varieties—high- and low-glycemic—are necessary for a rapid energy boost. Rapid insulin sensitivity brought on by high-glycemic carbs causes reactive hypoglycemia and tissue fat accumulation. Diets heavy in fat and sugar have the potential to inflame muscles, which are the primary site of glucose metabolism. Type 2 diabetes and insulin resistance may result from this inflammation.

The body uses starchy meals primarily for energy, but because processed foods lack fiber, consuming too much of them can elevate blood sugar levels more than whole grains do. Examples of these processed foods include white bread, rice, and pasta. The metabolic syndrome, which is characterized by insulin resistance, abnormal blood lipid levels, obesity, and elevated cholesterol, is closely associated with fructose consumption.

It is better to minimize or eliminate breads entirely to avoid these symptoms. While brown rice is tainted with arsenic, whole-grain breads are heavy in lectins, gluten, and glutamate. Quinoa, couscous, and farro are substitutes for white rice, but they have disadvantages and therefore to be avoided.

Sugar

The type of sugar affects how hazardous it is; glucose is less toxic than fructose.

This is the most recent research:

- Sugar is now considered the major cause of obesity, which leads not only to diabetes and heart disease, but is also implicated in other chronic ailments, including several types of cancer. Fructose is far more fattening than other sugars (especially high-fructose corn syrup).

- Sugar exacerbates inflammation and insulin resistance, which is the primary cause of atherosclerosis, heart attacks, strokes, neurological illnesses, and damage to other organs, including your liver! Once more, fructose is not as healthy for any of these illnesses as other sugars are.

- Regularly consuming excessive amounts of sugar can lead to reactive hypoglycemia in the end. Numerous health issues, including brain damage, may result from this.

- Dementia is associated with insulin resistance, which is brought on by fructose and sugar. Now known as "type 3 diabetes," this form of insulin resistance is thought to be present in Alzheimer's disease patients. It resembles the type 2 diabetes that most people are familiar with, but it seems to be isolated within the brain. Blood sugar can actually be absolutely normal outside of the brain. Furthermore, we are aware that elevated glucose levels are harmful to brain tissue, a phenomenon known as glucotoxicity.

- Because sugar is considered to be extremely addictive, your cravings for it will increase as you consume more of it.

Obesity, metabolic syndrome, neurodegenerative illnesses, reactive hypoglycemia, and inflammatory disorders are all significantly influenced by sugar. Refined sugar isn't the only type that is bad for you; raw, brown, honey, and molasses sugars also include healthy ingredients.

Artificial Sweeteners

Artificial sweeteners, especially those found in sodas, are bad for the liver because they can cause NAFLD, obesity, diabetes, and metabolic syndrome. Although stevia, a naturally occurring sweetener, may be good for the liver, it may also be harmful to brain and reproductive cells. An anti-inflammatory, non-nutritive sweetener that is healthy is monk fruit extract. Forty percent of Americans use toothpaste and prepackaged foods that contain sugar. Sugary foods make it harder to cut back on sugar intake because they activate brain receptors that cause insulin release.

Strategies for Sugar Reduction

- **Remove the blatant offenders**: Get rid of the soft drinks, candy, sugar bowl, and other items from your home, vehicle, and workplace!

- **Read labels carefully:** There are almost fifty names that sugar can go by. These are a few of the more typical ones. Lactose, brown rice syrup, molasses, dextrose, cane sugar, fructose, glucose, maltose, rice syrup, cane juice crystals, evaporated cane juice, raw sugar, organic raw sugar, maltodextrin, and many more can be found in the "ingredients" sections of various products.

- **Avoid purchasing any food items that include high-fructose corn syrup (HFCS):** This popular sweetener, found in sodas and fruit-flavored drinks, is produced in a manner that converts glucose into fructose, which is a sweeter form of sugar.

- **Make sure you're not just thirsty but truly hungry:** Cravings for sugar may indicate dehydration.

- **Get enough sleep:** Studies reveal that fatigued individuals often have a craving for junk food, particularly sugar. Suffering also intensifies the need for sweets.

- **Eliminate alcohol:** Alcohol and sweets both have an addictive quality. Cocktails are not only loaded with sugar, but drinking alcohol can make it easier to give up other sweets.

- **If you must have something sweet to satisfy your sweet craving, have a couple little squares of dark chocolate:** Compared to milk chocolate, which has additional sugar and fat, products with a larger percentage of dark chocolate have lower sugar contents.

Salt

Sodium chloride, sometimes referred to as salt, is necessary to keep fluid equilibrium. The majority of people consume more than the government-recommended daily allowance of less than 2,300 milligrams. Ten percent of the salt in food comes from natural sources, and the remaining five to ten percent comes from processed foods and food services. Heart disease, stroke, heart failure, and kidney disease can all be brought on by high blood pressure. Overindulgence in salt can exacerbate neurological conditions and have a direct impact on the liver, exacerbating metabolic syndrome and causing liver damage.

Here are some pointers to reduce your intake of salt:

- Use your saltshaker sparingly.

- **Eat whole, fresh foods:** Whenever feasible, choose foods that are organic. Processed and packaged foods are frequently laden with salt, which serves as a preservative in addition to flavor.

- **Learn to season meals without adding salt by using ingredients like lemon juice, black pepper, ginger, fennel, bay leaves, rosemary, ginger, and garlic:** When using salt alternatives, use caution because some of them contain potassium chloride, which is dangerous for those with kidney issues, or a blend of salt and other ingredients (referred to as "sodium" on labels). Therefore, you might wish to consult your physician first.

- **Never assume that sweets are devoid of salt:** Goods with a sweet taste, such cake mixes, sweets, and quick puddings, might all contain salt. Added to a lot of manufactured meals is salt.
- **Eliminate condiments:** Condiments like ketchup, barbeque sauce, meat tenderizers, and—most importantly—soy sauce frequently conceal salt.
- **Snack wisely:** Salt gives chips, pretzels, and crackers their flavor and addictive characteristic. Replace with fresh vegetables or, for a special treat, unsalted or reduced-sodium versions of your go-to foods.
- **Select fresh or frozen vegetables.:** Your best bet is to use fresh veggies. If unavailable, select frozen. Vegetables that are canned are frequently cooked with salt and even sugar.

- **Watch out for foods without fat or sugar:** Manufacturers typically use salt to replace components such as fat and sugar.

- **Don't follow very low-salt diets:** because they have the potential to produce significant salt depletion, which can result in serious disease and make it very difficult to safely recover the necessary salt level. These diets are commonly used to treat hypertension that is not well managed. Natural remedies for high blood pressure exist that are significantly safer, like hawthorn, Bonito fish extract, high-dose vitamin C, and Nano Grape Seed extract.

CHAPTER 5

Is Your Liver at Risk Due to Your Lifestyle?

The liver is essential for the detoxification and elimination of toxins from the environment and our bodies, such as alcohol, tobacco smoke, pollution, and tainted drinking water. Medical professionals inject, inhale, and absorb these drugs through the skin in addition to ingesting them. Adopting a healthier lifestyle can help prevent conditions like renal disease, high blood pressure, diabetes, cancer, heart disease, stroke, chronic lung disease, gastrointestinal disorders, and neurodegenerative illnesses. Boosting the detoxification of the liver also boosts the detoxification of cells.

Smoking

More than 4,000 toxic compounds are released when smoking, and these chemicals can have a negative impact on the liver, arteries, brain, and other organs. It is an extremely inflammatory and potentially fatal condition that produces free radicals. A lifetime smoker's chances of dying from tobacco-related causes are 50%, and their average lifespan is only 10 years. In addition to respiratory disorders, smokers are more likely to develop chronic illnesses such as liver damage. Studies reveal a connection between smoking and faster disease progression in individuals suffering from fatty liver disease, alcoholic liver disease, and chronic hepatitis C and B. Additionally, smoking raises the risk of liver cancer, however the risk is lower in former smokers than in current smokers. Because nicotine in tobacco smoke is a potent immune system suppressant, it raises the risk of liver infections and certain malignancies, including brain tumors. While e-cigarettes may seem like a healthier option, they can lead to long-term hypoxia, serious lung damage, and the buildup of hazardous elements like propylene glycol in the liver, which raises the risk of both liver damage and brain cancer.

Alcohol Use

Because alcohol is absorbed in the digestive tract and metabolized in the liver to produce toxic chemicals, drinking alcohol is bad for the liver. Three forms of liver injury are caused by overindulgence: cirrhosis, fat buildup, and fat accumulation.

The following illnesses are directly related to consuming excessive amounts of alcohol:

- **Fat accumulation (hepatic steatosis):** Liver fat might develop as a result of excessive alcohol consumption. Over 90% of individuals who consume excessive amounts of alcohol experience this; nevertheless, it is typically reversible upon stopping drinking. Binge drinking, or consuming huge amounts of alcohol quickly, can cause a fatty liver to grow quickly. In rare situations, it can even cause catastrophic liver destruction and result in death within minutes, especially if the person already has liver problems.

- **Alcoholic hepatitis:** This is the kind of hepatitis that is caused by alcohol consumption. The word "hepatitis" signifies inflammation. The most common cause of alcoholic hepatitis is heavy drinking over a period of years. The association between drinking and this illness is not always evident—sometimes big drinkers do not get this illness, and other times it can strike non-drinkers as well. It is estimated that between 10 and 35 percent of chronic heavy drinkers suffer with this illness. The extent of alcohol-induced toxic damage is contingent upon an individual's nutritional state, particularly with regard to the consumption of water-soluble vitamins like folate, vitamin B12, and the B-complex. These vitamins provide the liver with a great deal of protection.

- **Cirrhosis:** Chronic heavy drinkers have a 10–20% chance of developing cirrhosis, a potentially fatal disease where scar tissue replaces healthy liver cells. Liver cells cannot be replaced by scar tissue. The liver eventually gets smaller. In contrast to alcoholic hepatitis and fatty liver, severe cirrhosis is irreversible.

When alcohol is ingested in excess of 1.5 ounces per day for more than ten years, liver damage may result. Libido sensitivity to alcohol damage is increased when alcohol is combined with hazardous medications such as Tylenol or prescription drugs. Glutathione, the body's primary defense molecule, starts to diminish around age 40 and guards against viral infections. When alcohol is consumed empty-handed, its hazardous effects are amplified. Wine's composition varies from brand to brand, but it always contains good stuff from grapes that shield the liver. The majority of wines have high concentrations of harmful fluoride and sulfites. High concentrations of lectins, gluten, and aluminum found in beer can damage cells and exacerbate arthritis. Because aluminum can leach out of acidic cans and kegs, there may be a risk.

Men and women can both get liver damage from alcohol, but women are more susceptible because of their smaller bodies. Males are better at clearing alcohol from their systems than women are, but over 0.75 to 1.5 ounces a day puts women at risk. Since alcohol is more susceptible to hepatic impairment or underlying disorders, abstinence is the only recommended course of action.

Obesity

Because of inflammation, increased risk of diabetes, hypertension, depression, brain diseases, atherosclerosis, infections, and metabolic syndromes, being overweight is hazardous. According to recent studies, eating too much may set off the immune system, resulting in persistent inflammation of the body and harm to internal organs, including the liver. When visceral fat builds up in the abdomen, the body and liver experience severe inflammation. Nonalcoholic fatty liver disease (NAFLD) and nonalcoholic steatohepatitis (NASH), which can damage the liver and perhaps result in primary liver cancer, are also caused by obesity and overweight.

Toxic Food Dyes

Colorful food dyes, some of which have been found to be harmful, are common. Manufacturers are permitted by the FDA to perform their own safety testing; nevertheless, numerous manufacturers alter these tests to conceal negative consequences. Red 40, Yellow 5, and Yellow 6 are the most often used dyes and are found in beverages, dessert powders, baked products, sweets, cereals, and prescription medications. Children consume more than the recommended safe amounts, and as China lacks strict food safety laws, a large number of these dyes are currently imported. These dyes are particularly hazardous to children since they are consumed in larger doses than by adults. All things considered, no one should eat food or use medication that contains these dyes.

Exposure to Herbicides, Fungicides, and Pesticides

It has been discovered that chemical pesticides and weed killers have detrimental health impacts, especially to infants, young children, and teenagers. It has been demonstrated that even at low dosages, a class of pesticides known as organophosphorus insecticides can harm the developing brains of infants, neonates, and teenagers. Researchers have also discovered that male progeny subjected to the common organic pesticide chlorpyrifos exhibit higher hostility. These substances harm the liver, resulting in abnormal liver enzyme levels, increased inflammation, and cell death. Schools are regularly exposed to these harmful substances as well. Parkinson's, ALS, and Alzheimer's disease have all been related to pesticide and herbicide exposure. According to research conducted by the U.S. Geological Survey, thirty percent of these chemicals' breakdown products in the environment are more hazardous than the original molecule. Herbicides, especially those containing glyphosate, have been discovered in a variety of locations, including playgrounds, public buildings, houses, offices, meals, drinks, lakes, streams, and groundwater.

CHAPTER 6

Artificial Sweeteners and Food Additives

The liver is required to detoxify or metabolize the harmful substances included in processed meals, beverages, and soups since they are alien to the human body. Particularly when combined, many of these substances have never undergone sufficient testing to ensure their long-term safety. When combined, the chemicals' synergistic toxicity is increased. Processed foods and beverages abound in most stores, and more are on the horizon. Manufactured meats and "meat glue," which is gluing less expensive slices of meat together using special enzymes and harmful excitotoxins, are examples of modern food advancements. Although statistics indicate that we are living longer, this trend appears to be coming to an end. The prevalence of degenerative disorders, including multiple sclerosis, ALS, Alzheimer's dementia, Parkinson's disease, and seizures, is increasing. This trend is attributed to microwave radiation and Wi-Fi usage. Inadequate testing has been done on chemical food additives, household items, industrial chemicals, vaccinations, and agricultural chemicals. These chemicals might intensify the negative consequences of an unhealthful diet.

Excitotoxins

The liver performs a herculean role in feeding and shielding the body, but toxic exposures from outside sources in today's contemporary life harm it in numerous ways. Eating large amounts of these excitotoxic food additives is one of the frequently disregarded ways we are damaging our own health. Excitotoxins are added to most processed foods in one or more forms.

Glutamate receptors in the brain control neuronal excitement, but they are also harmful to the brain. Increased quantities of glutamate outside of cells lead to autoimmune disorders, meningitis, convulsions, stroke, neurodegenerative illnesses, and brain damage. Overindulgence in dietary additives containing excitotoxins can penetrate the brain and aggravate certain conditions. Since almost all cells have glutamate receptors, eating foods high in carbohydrates, such as MSG and aspartame, can harm every organ and tissue in the body. Most diseases are caused by excitotoxins because they exacerbate lipid peroxidation, inflammation, and the production of free radicals.

Liver disorders and excitotoxins

Animals who consume an excessive amount of glutamate may develop fatty liver disease and cirrhosis as a result of liver inflammation and cell damage. Pregnant animals exposed to MSG may experience changes in the liver's hepatic metabolization of lipids, leading to increased levels of cholesterol and other fats linked to disease. Consuming high-fructose corn syrup—in particular, high-fructose corn syrup—has a strong correlation with cirrhosis and fatty liver disease. Consuming high-fructose foods along with MSG affects the liver and increases visceral fat, which raises the risk of heart attacks and strokes. MSG has the potential to prolong liver inflammation, which raises the risk of primary liver cancer and cirrhosis. Elevated fructose and glutamate food additives cause persistent inflammation in the liver, increasing the risk of fatty liver diseases, especially in young children. High dietary glutamate intake and high fructose corn syrup intake exacerbate liver-damaging processes and raise the risk of primary liver cancer.

Concealing Excitotoxin Additives in Processed Foods

Brain damage and unpleasant reactions like the Chinese restaurant syndrome have been connected to monosodium glutamate (MSG). When Dr. John Olney discovered that consuming MSG damages the brain, the practice of adding MSG to baby food was discontinued. Food processors' entrenched interests in the multimillion-dollar sector made them hesitant to remove MSG. Instead of using high-glutamate additions, they covered up the identities of glutamate-containing food additives. Food processors were permitted by regulatory bodies to use deceptive labels, like "Contains no MSG," even if their ingredients comprised a high concentration of glutamate. It's critical to study food labels, stay away from processed meals, and prioritize fresh, organic foods in order to prevent glutamate food additives.

Cheaper slices of meat are joined to resemble more expensive cuts using meat glues, a novel source of glutamate excitotoxins. High glutamate content chemicals give produced foods the flavor profile of more expensive meats. Maybe even more dangerous than MSG are these glues.

The following are a some of the most widely used code names for food additives high in glutamate:

- Monosodium glutamate
- Hydrolyzed vegetable protein
- Hydrolyzed protein
- Hydrolyzed plant protein
- Plant protein extract
- Sodium caseinate
- Calcium caseinate

- Yeast extract

- Textured protein

- Autolyzed yeast

- Hydrolyzed oat flour

- Soy protein concentrate

- Protein concentrate

- Carrageenan enzymes (Protease enzymes from various sources can

- release excitotoxin amino acids from food proteins.)

The following additives almost always contain MSG:

- Malt extract

- Malt flavoring

- Bouillon broth

- Stock flavoring

- Natural flavoring

- Natural beef- or chicken-flavored seasoning spices

- Seasoning spices

Trans Fats, MSG, and Fatty Liver Disease

In one study, Dr. Collison and her associates looked at the effects of eating a diet heavy in trans fats along with MSG. Excessive trans fats have been connected to heart disease, insulin resistance, and obesity. The deadliest type of fat, visceral fat, can be increased by MSG and trans fats, according to the research. The rats were given a diet heavy in trans fats, a mild dose of MSG, or a combination of the two. High levels of triglycerides and free fatty acids were the result of the combination, which is associated with an increased risk of cardiovascular illnesses.

Aspartame

Common artificial sweetener aspartame is metabolized to produce methanol and formaldehyde, which is a hazardous substance that attaches itself securely to proteins and damages DNA over time. Aspartame and MSG together can raise visceral and liver fat, which raises the risk of conditions such degenerative brain disorders, heart disease, liver failure, and sleep apnea. In addition to raising blood sugar, insulin resistance, and inflammation, combining MSG, aspartame, and trans fats can also increase inflammation and the risk of type 2 diabetes. When consuming them together, it is imperative to stay away from these dangerous chemicals.

Animals who consume aspartame on a regular basis have been shown to have severe liver and kidney damage. The adverse effects include low glutathione levels, high lipid peroxidation, and nitric oxide. Nitric oxide can be extremely inflammatory and excitotoxic, despite being an essential molecule for cell protection. Animals given aspartame daily for two to six weeks see a rise in liver lipid peroxidation as well as a decrease in vital antioxidant enzymes such as glutathione, catalase, and superoxide dismutase. Because of this, the liver is more susceptible to harmful substances, which raises the possibility of severe liver disease or liver cancer. We are more at danger from aspartame and excitotoxic food additives like MSG than from keeping our livers healthy.

Sodas account for over 70% of all aspartame consumption. It's also used to sweeten a lot of drugs, particularly kids' medications. It ought to have been outlawed when it was first suggested, in my opinion. There was ample proof that the FDA was persuaded to allow this harmful sweetener even though it was obvious that it was far too risky to use as a sweetener. It is necessary to fix this error.

Comparing Saccharin with Aspartame

A dangerous chemical connected to a number of cancers is aspartame. When its toxicity was compared to saccharin, a study discovered that saccharin was even more harmful. Increased enzymes, histopathological damage, and liver damage were all brought on by these sweeteners. At comparable concentrations, saccharin damaged DNA more than aspartame.

Avoidance of Aspartame Toxicity

A number of organs, including the liver, kidneys, heart, reproductive system, and brain, can sustain serious harm from aspartame. By increasing the amounts of antioxidant enzymes and correcting glutathione suppression, natural substances like L-carnitine can dramatically minimize damage. Aspartame damage can be prevented by selenium, but daily doses should be kept to a minimum. Significant protection against liver damage is provided by naturally occurring compounds that inhibit oxidative stress, such as R-lipoic acid, NAC, Nano-Curcumin, Nano-Quercetin, and Nano-Silymarin.

CHAPTER 7

Steer Clear of Liver-Toxic Chemicals

Merely one percent of the food supply is screened for dangerous ingredients, according to a new analysis of the regulatory procedure. Every minute of every day, we are subjected to tens of thousands of industrial toxins, drinking water additives, microwave radiation, and other dangerous impacts. Toxicity may be multiplied by synergistic toxicity.

When weak carcinogens, pesticides, herbicides, and fungicides are combined, they can cause synergistic toxicity, which can result in cancer. There is a dearth of safety testing for these harmful chemicals; the majority of studies are short-term and do not examine long-term consequences. Because harmful substances can persist for months, years, or even lifetimes, bioaccumulation is another issue. Since some pesticides are systemic and cannot be removed by washing, we should refrain from contaminating veggies with veggie washes in order to protect ourselves. Vegetables and some meats, such as tomatoes, cattle, potatoes, celery, kale, lettuce, oranges, apples, peaches, pig, wheat, soybeans, carrots, chicken, corn, and grapes, have the highest concentration of pesticides.

The toxicity of more than 65,000 chemicals, especially those that affect the nervous system, has not been sufficiently studied, according to the Environmental Protection Agency's registry. Tens of millions of individuals have several of these chemicals in their homes, and over nine million people have frequent contact with neurotoxins at work. Every year, more than a thousand new compounds are added, the majority of which have undergone inadequate testing. Additionally, the chemical industry uses two million blends, mixes, and other formulations, of which over 60,000 are known to cause brain damage. There are 64 pesticides that have been found to have the potential to cause cancer worldwide. Farm workers are more likely to suffer from neurological problems and malignancies.

Research indicates that cats and kids who live in yards that use pesticides are more likely to develop leukemia. Each year, illnesses linked to pesticides impact between 150,000 and 500,000 people, resulting in 200 fatalities and numerous other seriously injured people. In order to avoid or lessen these negative effects, the condition of our detoxification systems, particularly the liver, is essential. Aspartame is one example of a chemical that damages the liver and can hinder detoxification and make you more vulnerable to harmful drugs.

Toxic substances and endocrine disruptors

Endocrine disruptors, which persist in the environment and cause diseases, include pesticides, herbicides, fungicides, and PCBs. They are also present in common compounds including phthalates, bisphenol A, dioxins, and insecticides.

Phthalates

Every person in the United States has some amount of the industrial chemical's phthalates in their bodies, which have polluted the environment. Lower molecular forms are utilized in lacquers, varnishes, coatings, and personal care products, whereas high molecular weight forms are used as plasticizers in the production of PVC.

Phthalates are anti-androgens that have been associated with aberrant development of the male but not the female sexual organs during pregnancy. There is a clear correlation between exposure to phthalates and aberrant development of male reproductive organs, according to a major study involving 737 newborns. The problem is attributed to very modest concentrations of phthalates.

Complexes of Fluoride and Fluor Aluminum

Dental goods and treatments frequently contain aluminum and fluoride, which are present in drinking water. There is no scientific evidence to support the mandates of state governors and city governments to introduce them to public drinking water systems. Fluoride weakens dental enamel, according to studies, which raises the incidence of cavities and dental fluorosis.

Many foods and beverages contain fluoride and aluminum, with black tea having the highest concentrations of both metals. Aluminum is widely available and can be found in foil, baking powder, trays, cups, canned goods, and aluminum cookware. They combine to create a toxic fluor aluminum complex that can harm organs and tissues. Aluminum has been connected to neurological conditions such as ALS and Alzheimer's disease. Because fluor aluminum kills liver cells, particularly those involved in detoxification, the liver is the first organ to be affected by poisoning. Fluor aluminum complexes are better absorbed from the gastrointestinal tract than aluminum alone, which is poorly absorbed.

Substances that were outlawed in 2000 are still present in the environment and can harm the kidneys and liver. According to research on animals, they can harm the liver and cause cancer, damage to the reproductive system, and brain impairment. Use respirator masks, high-speed room ventilation, and lower-aluminum and fluoride white or green tea to reduce these dangers. Select foods and water that have been filtered or distillated organically.

Protecting Your Liver

Natural ingredients such as saffron, taurine, and nano-curcumin can be used to protect the liver from toxins and improve detoxification. Organophosphate pesticide toxicity is decreased by saffron, and rotenone and chlorpyrifos are better detoxified by taurine and nano-curcumin. Rotenone toxicity is lessened by other substances such as Triphala, blueberry extract, and nano-grape seed extract. Other substances, such as baicalin, L-carnitine, and R-lipoic acid, have been demonstrated to prevent advanced cirrhosis patients from losing their minds and becoming confused, lower visceral fat and fatty liver disease, and inhibit muscle loss. Additionally, natural substances that offer protection against fatty liver disease include R-lipoic acid, NAC, B-complex vitamins, myo-inositol, trans-ferulic acid, and pterostilbene. It has been demonstrated that taurine, an amino acid that contains sulfur, prevents liver fibrosis and other liver damage.

CHAPTER 8

The Liver Poisoning Effects of Drugs

Although the pharmaceuticals you take may help your body, your liver plays a major role in the metabolization of these substances, which can lead to damage to the liver. When allergic reactions and overdoses are taken out of the picture, drug responses cause between 100,000 and 300,000 deaths per year. The four-step "ADME" process—an abbreviation for absorption, distribution, metabolism, and excretion—is how the body processes medications. Administered medications enter the bloodstream and reach their destination through the bloodstream after being taken orally, intravenously, or by injection. These medications are metabolized by the liver, where enzymes and other metabolic processes change some of the chemicals.

When medications directly damage the liver's cells, they limit the liver's ability to detoxify and metabolize substances, leading to liver toxicity, hepatic toxicity, or toxic hepatitis. Even at recommended dosages, this can result in harmful substances. Compared to natural items, pharmaceutical medications are more dangerous and rarely result in death.

Liver damage can take many different forms, ranging from a slight increase in liver enzymes to severe liver failure. Liver injury that is mild to moderate is mostly 100% reparable. The result of acute liver failure is contingent upon the toxic material to which the patient is exposed. For instance, most patients who receive prompt treatment for acetaminophen poisoning—even those with abrupt liver failure—will fully recover. When using other drugs, the liver does not heal and the patient has hepatic encephalopathy, which quickly results in a coma and death.

Of all the organs and tissues in the body, the liver possesses one of the most amazing capacities for regeneration. It is frequently possible to heal even severe liver damage, particularly with the use of specific antioxidants and naturally occurring anti-inflammatory substances. The following elements put you at risk for liver damage caused by toxins:

- Being age 65 or older
- Being female
- Taking more over-the-counter pain relievers than the recommended dose
- Taking over-the-counter pain relievers, or certain medications or supplements with alcohol
- Combining one or more liver toxic substances at the same time (drug synergy)
- Chronic use of artificial sweeteners that are known to be liver toxic such as aspartame
- Having an underlying liver condition, such as cirrhosis, fatty liver disease, or hepatitis
- Working or having worked in a job that uses industrial chemicals that can damage the liver

Symptoms of Toxic Liver Disease

- Unexplained fever
- Diarrhea
- Dark-colored urine
- Itching
- Jaundice, or yellowish eyes and skin
- Headaches
- Loss of appetite
- Nausea
- Stomach pain or pain on the upper right-hand side of the abdomen
- Vomiting
- Weight loss
- White or gray stool

Some Drugs that Cause Liver Toxicity

- Acetaminophen (Tylenol)
- Amoxicillin/clavulanate (Augmentin)
- Diclofenac (Voltaren, Cambia)
- Amiodarone (Cordarone, Pacerone)
- Allopurinol (Zyloprim)
- Antiseizure medications
- Methotrexate

- Statins (cholesterol-lowering medication)
- Antipsychotic medications

Acetaminophen (Tylenol)

In both the US and the UK, acetaminophen overdoses account for 20% of liver transplants and 450 fatalities per year due to acute liver failure. Since taking numerous drugs containing acetaminophen can increase vulnerability, unintentional intoxication is more common than purposeful poisoning. In addition to depleting liver glutathione levels, starvation diets, fasting, and chronic alcohol use can further increase a person's risk of acetaminophen poisoning. Aspartame, an artificial sweetener, can also severely deplete hepatic glutathione, increasing a person's risk of acetaminophen intoxication. Usually starting within 24 hours, symptoms progress through four stages before severe liver failure occurs. Glutathione levels are quickly raised by taking N-acetyl-L-cysteine, which is the treatment. Nonetheless, a deadly allergy to the sulfur component of NAC can occur in certain individuals. Acetaminophen liver damage can also be inhibited by natural substances such as trans-ferulic acid, luteolin, apigenin, hesperidin, baicalin, hesperidin, trans-curcumin, and nano-quercetin.

Antibiotics

Antibiotics are administered frequently to maintain blood levels and treat infections because they are processed in the liver. Drug levels may be prolonged by detoxification-related issues, particularly in individuals with liver conditions like cirrhosis. A few antibiotics can harm the liver, including erythromycin, amoxicillin/clavulanic acid, flucloxacillin, azithromycin, chloramphenicol, and lincomycin. Fluoroquinolones, a class of newly developed antibiotics, have a fluorine component that inhibits detoxification and prolongs the drug's half-life at greater dosages. These fluoride antibiotics are linked to suicidal thoughts and homicidal impulses, and they also have a greater likelihood of complications. Educating physicians about natural chemicals and their possible toxicity is essential.

Arthritis Drugs

When rheumatoid arthritis patients take methotrexate or azathioprine, liver damage is frequently reported. Methotrexate releases adenosine, which inhibits molecules that promote inflammation, slowing the progression of the disease and relieving its symptoms. One person out of every 1000 will experience liver damage as a result of using methotrexate. The second most prevalent cause of drug-induced liver injury is non-steroidal anti-inflammatory medicines (NSAIDs), which are more hazardous when combined with metabolic syndrome and fatty liver disorders. Rheumatoid arthritis is one example of an autoimmune disease that makes the liver more susceptible to all of the drugs used to treat it. When paired with pharmaceutical medications for arthritis, natural anti-inflammatory substances like Nano-Curcumin, Nano-Silymarin, L-carnitine, and baicalin can improve the efficacy and safety of the former.

Antifungal Drugs

Doctors should keep an eye on liver functions when using antifungal medications since they can harm the liver, particularly if there is underlying liver disease. Different medications can cause different levels of liver damage. While azole classes cause minor damage but can result in fatal failure, flucytosine can induce damage to the liver. Micafungin carries a caution for people with liver illness because it can cause liver tumors when processed by enzymes other than P-450 phase I.

Steroids

Furthermore, corticosteroids have a significant impact on the liver, especially when used over an extended period of time and at doses above what is advised. They can also cause or exacerbate nonalcoholic steatohepatitis (NASH), a more severe kind of fatty liver disease. The use of glucocorticoids may cause the liver to expand and store fat. However, these medications have shown excellent results when used to treat autoimmune liver disease and liver failure brought on by viral hepatitis.

Corticosteroids have the potential to save lives when used for such circumstances, usually in the short term. Furthermore, corticosteroids have a significant impact on the liver, especially when used over an extended period of time and at doses above what is advised. They can also cause or exacerbate nonalcoholic steatohepatitis (NASH), a more severe kind of fatty liver disease. The use of glucocorticoids may cause the liver to expand and store fat. However, these medications have shown excellent results when used to treat autoimmune liver disease and liver failure brought on by viral hepatitis. Corticosteroids have the potential to save lives when used for such circumstances, usually in the short term.

Antiseizure Medications

Drugs used to treat epilepsy, such as carbamazepine and Dilantin, can harm the liver and result in seizures. It's crucial to talk to your doctor about using medications for epilepsy. Altering one's diet and using natural substances like myoinositol, magnesium, taurine, baicalin, nano-Bacopa, nano-

Curcumin, and nano-Ashwagandha are safer options. These organic substances not only prevent seizures but also enhance overall health, which includes liver function. Before using these drugs, speak with your doctor.

Psychotropic Medications

Liver damage can result from antidepressants, mood stabilizers, anxiety reducers, and antipsychotics. Hepatotoxic drugs include tricyclic antidepressants, antipsychotics, and mood stabilizers such as lamotrigine, valproate, topiramate, and carbamazepine. These medications occasionally cause liver damage, particularly in people who already have liver disease.

Statins

The production and distribution of cholesterol, which is required for many physiological processes and utilized by the brain, are mostly controlled by the liver. The myth that high cholesterol causes atherosclerosis and heart attacks served as the foundation for the marketing of statin cholesterol-lowering medications. New research, however, indicates that tiny dense LDL cholesterol is the sole type of cholesterol that causes atherosclerosis and is associated with risk. Because of their dose-related side effects, statins, such as atorvastatin, Fluvastatin, lovastatin, Pitavastatin, pravastatin, rosuvastatin, and simvastatin, are linked to liver and muscle damage.

CHAPTER 9

Liver and the Adrenal Gland

Situated above the kidneys, the adrenal glands release vital chemicals that are necessary for the body to operate. They generate the hormones that control the immune system, blood pressure, metabolism, and stress reaction. The majority of adrenal issues are related to endocrine processes, especially those involving steroids like cortisone. The link between the adrenal gland and the liver is complicated. Adrenal insufficiency affects 33% of people with liver illness, which frequently results in adrenal dysfunction. Poor adrenal gland function is a common consequence of chronic liver failure; in fact, 95% of patients undergoing liver transplantation had under functioning adrenal glands. Liver damage is also linked to other endocrine disorders like diabetes and underactive thyroid.

Gallbladder Disease

Bile is stored in the gallbladder, a little sac located beneath the liver, and then sent to the small intestine for digestion. In the United States, 20–25 million people suffer from gallbladder disease, a chronic gastrointestinal ailment that is most frequent in Native Americans (20–25 million). Pregnancy, obesity, fast weight loss, liver cirrhosis, hemolytic anemia, being a woman, and certain drugs are risk factors. In Western nations, cholesterol is the cause of 75-80% of gallstones. The development of cholesterol stones is exacerbated by gallbladder bacteria and poor motility. Gallstones are less common when magnesium lowers inflammation. Turmeric extracts, such as curcumin, have anti-inflammatory and antibacterial qualities, stimulate the gallbladder's contraction, and protect the liver against gallstones.

Obesity and Liver Disease

Obesity raises the risk of several illnesses, including diabetes, neurological diseases, heart attacks, heart failure, atherosclerosis, strokes, and some malignancies. Visceral obesity, in particular, is commonly referred to as having a "beer gut." Additionally linked to liver problems, obesity makes these conditions worse by accelerating their progression and widening their scope.

Fatty livers are associated with a 4.6-fold rise in obesity, and the incidence is higher in whites, blacks, and Hispanics. Fatty liver disease (NAFLD) and obesity are closely associated with insulin resistance, which is a compromised cellular response to insulin. However, liver enzyme tests, which can be unreliable, are the primary method used by clinicians to screen patients for liver issues. Assessing fatty liver disease is better done with ultrasonography. The risk of developing advanced cirrhosis or liver cancer increases when benign fatty liver disease (BFL) progresses to inflammatory liver disease (NASH), which can be caused by delays in diagnosis. Blood triglyceride levels that are elevated along with obesity and insulin resistance are indicators of a high risk of liver fibrosis. Regarding the likelihood of developing cirrhosis and liver cancer, obesity combined with hidden early cirrhosis is equivalent to having hepatitis C.

CHAPTER 10

Diabetes and The Liver

Diabetes, or diabetes mellitus, is the seventh largest cause of death in the United States and is associated with a number of serious conditions, including as kidney disease, heart disease, nerve damage, blindness, and amputations. It interferes with the body's capacity to use glucose, severely harming organs and tissues. Acute liver failure, cirrhosis, liver fibrosis, liver cancer, and fatty liver disease (NAFLD and NASH) are all significantly influenced by diabetes. Pre-diabetes is associated with insulin resistance and the metabolic syndrome, and it is on the rise worldwide, notably in the United States. There are two types of diabetes:

- insulin dependent or juvenile diabetes.
- insulin resistant (glucose intolerance) diabetes.

A major contributing factor to the obesity, metabolic syndrome, and type 2 diabetes epidemic is the extensive usage of high-fructose corn syrup.

Treating liver disorders that have progressed requires strict control over insulin sensitivity.

How Common Is Diabetes?

Since 1980, the number of Americans with type 2 diabetes has tripled, accounting for 29 million people or 8% of the total population. Pre-diabetes affects about 86 million people; early changes are frequently missed. Type 2 diabetes affects one in ten persons worldwide, and since 1980, the percentage has more than doubled.

What Is the Liver's Role?

Diabetes is a metabolic disease that damages cells, tissues, and organs by impairing the body's capacity to metabolize blood glucose. Glucotoxicity, or too much sugar, can contaminate the brain. Natural glucose production occurs in the liver and kidneys, with the liver also producing and storing glycogen and breaking down proteins and lipids into sugars. To avoid stressing the pancreas' ability to generate insulin, which could lead to the death of insulin-producing cells, the liver releases glucose in little amounts. This may cause type 2 diabetes to become type 1 diabetes, requiring frequent injections of insulin. The relationship between fatty liver disease and diabetes provides more evidence of the liver's influence on the pancreas.

Type 2 Diabetes: Diabetes's Most Common Type

The most prevalent type of diabetes, type 2, affects 90–95% of cases. It is typified by high insulin and blood sugar levels because of damaged insulin receptors on cell surfaces. Insulin resistance results from this, which raises insulin and glucose levels over time. Diabetes is becoming more common as a result of poor diet, inactivity, and obesity. Inflammation, harm to blood vessels, retinas, the brain, kidneys, and heart can all result from insulin resistance. Additionally, it promotes the buildup of fat, especially visceral fat, which has a strong correlation with inflammation and insulin resistance.

Symptoms of Type 2 Diabetes

- Being hungry after eating

- Feeling tired frequently
- Being very thirsty
- Urinating often
- Losing weight without reason
- Numbness in the hands or feet
- Blurry vision
- Sores that heal very slowly

Type 2 diabetes, sometimes known as "silent diabetes" or pre-diabetes, can develop gradually and cause serious harm to the body, especially the liver. Early symptoms may manifest earlier than previously believed.

What Is Insulin Resistance?

Pre-diabetes, another name for early-stage insulin resistance, is a silent precursor to diabetes. In other words, as soon as symptoms start to show up, you have a warning sign alerting you to the fact you have a very high chance of getting diabetes if you don't modify your lifestyle, especially by losing weight and eating differently. The good news is that altering one's diet, losing weight, and using various natural flavonoid products can all help to reverse insulin resistance. More recent research is demonstrating that natural substances extracted from particular plants, including berberine, can treat insulin resistance and stop the harm this condition causes.

Causes of Diabetes?

The main cause of type 2 diabetes is obesity. Having excess weight increases the risk of developing diabetes. Although this is particularly true if diabetes runs in your family, obesity increases risk even in the absence of genetics, thus gaining weight in middle age increases your risk even if no family members have the condition. This holds true even if you simply gain a modest amount of weight in your middle years; nevertheless, your risk increases as you gain more weight. Once more, visceral fat—as opposed to subcutaneous fat, which is stored beneath the skin—is the most significant form of weight gain. As previously noted, a number of plant flavonoids have the ability to specifically reduce visceral fat, increasing the likelihood that your diabetes and even metabolic syndrome will be resolved.

Diabetes Treatment?

The primary treatment for diabetes is lowering blood sugar levels using food, oral drugs, or insulin. Additionally, routine screening for problems is necessary. Previously thought to be incurable, type 2 diabetes can now be prevented and even reversed with consistent exercise, a nutritious diet, the use of plant flavonoids and other unique natural chemicals, and weight loss. That message hasn't reached many doctors, though, and many lack the skills necessary to properly assist patients in changing their lifestyles.

Type 2 Diabetes Is Reversible!

According to research that was published in the Lancet, people with type 2 diabetes who have had the condition for less than six years may still be able to reverse it. In this trial, around 300 participants were randomized to follow their usual treatment and diet plans or participate in a weight control program. 46% of the diet group's participants reversed their diabetes, according to the results, suggesting that even people with a diagnosis of the full-blown condition may be able to do so.

Diabetics experience several dangerous side effects, such as:

- Blindness
- Cataracts
- Impotence in men
- Kidney failure
- Rapid atherosclerosis (amputation of limbs)
- Heart failure
- Strokes
- Liver failure
- Dysbiosis (an imbalance in the gut bacteria)
- Neurodegenerative diseases
- Peripheral neuropathy
- Muscle loss
- Pulmonary disorders
- Frequent infections (immune suppression)
- Increased cancer rates

Tips on Weight Loss

As you've seen, one of the keys in reversing diabetes is weight loss. Here are some tips:

Fruits and Vegetables

The Rule Is Moderation Fruits should only be consumed in moderation because they differ in their sugar content. Some people gain weight when they are around sugar. Whole fruits should be avoided, but fruit extracts with the sugar removed can be used. Less sugar and modest levels of better-tolerated complex carbohydrates can be found in vegetables. Vegetables are important because they include various flavonoid components that lower lipid peroxidation, a major issue associated with diabetes, and damage caused by free radicals. If consumed in moderation, complex carbs (only when consumed in small amounts) allow the body to gradually convert them into glucose and avoid fat gain.

Eat Protein in Moderation

For several reasons, animal protein is essential to overall health. Animals fed organic food should provide the majority of your protein needs. Recent research has demonstrated that the warnings issued by numerous health organizations regarding the risks associated with eating meat are untrue and that meats raised organically contain balanced proteins, healthy oils, and flavonoids—consistencies that naturally occur in fruits and vegetables—that are essential for overall health. Meats that are not raised organically are higher in industrial chemicals, fungicides, herbicides, and pesticides (which are concentrated in the fats) and can exacerbate the effects of diabetes. Because the majority of cattle populations have viruses that might cause cancer and neurological disorders in their tissues, beef shouldn't be consumed raw. Researchers discovered cancer-causing viruses in 80% of the animals they looked at in some herds. These viruses are killed by heat, yet they can live in rare-cooked foods. Research has demonstrated that even those who handle raw meats at slaughterhouses have a markedly increased risk of hemopoietic malignancies, such as multiple myeloma, lymphoma, and leukemia.

Fiber: The Positive and Negative

High-fiber foods, such as various fruits and vegetables (preferably organic, even with the skins on), have two advantages for you: They will first make you feel fuller and less hungry. They also lower the risk of colon cancer. Soluble fiber is especially advantageous. Citrus fruits, chicory, strawberries, oat bran, and inulin are excellent providers of soluble fiber. The bacteria in the colon eat soluble fiber. Research has demonstrated that grain fiber does not prevent cancer; only vegetable fiber does. Some sources of fiber are as follows:

Legumes

Some of the greatest foods to eat for soluble fiber are beans, peas, and almonds. Beans are satiating and high in protein. Some good sources of antioxidants are beans. All beans should be cooked all the way through due to the high quantities of lectins that can be harmful to your health. Certain beans, like black beans, also contain a lot of the excitotoxin glutamate. Excitotoxins can harm the liver, particularly a diseased liver, and they can also promote the growth of malignancies.

Brussels sprouts and broccoli

Soluble fiber may be found in a variety of vegetables, and broccoli and Brussels sprouts are among the best. (Asparagus and sweet potatoes are also delicious.) They must be cooked thoroughly because they contain a lot of lectins, much like the beans. You should cook them in water or by steaming them. Both have strong anticancer effects, safeguard the cardiovascular system, protect the brain, and are rich in antioxidant flavonoids.

Blueberries and other berries.

Numerous health benefits, such as anticancer capabilities, cardiac blood vessel health, and prevention of brain aging, are associated with berries including blackberries, strawberries, and raspberries. Strawberries and blueberries have an ingredient called senolytic that slows down the aging process. Oranges and other citrus fruits have a high soluble fiber content, but because of their high sugar content, they should only be eaten in moderation. The most potent ingredients are concentrated in sugar-free blueberry extract capsules. The liver-protecting compound pterostilbene is more readily absorbed than resveratrol.

Use Olive Oil

The author recommends using premium, cold-pressed extra virgin olive oil in place of saturated or trans fats, such as butter or margarine. Margarine, which is toxic and encourages the growth of cancer, is made from oxidized omega-6 oil. Olive oil protects the brain, lowers the risk of cancer, stops blood clotting, and brings blood sugar levels back to normal. The anticancer and antioxidant properties of turmeric can be strengthened.

Avoid All Dairy Products

Dairy products have been linked to several health issues, such as a higher risk of heart attacks and strokes. Actually, research indicates that the risk of heart attacks is increased while drinking low-fat milk as opposed to full milk. Cow's milk is on the list of foods frequently linked to allergies and is also significantly related with juvenile diabetes. Due to its high calcium and glutamate content, milk promotes the proliferation of cancer cells.

Steer clear of breads, biscuits, and anything made with rye, barley, or wheat.

A common grain, gluten, has been connected to neurological conditions like autism and neurodegeneration. Avoid all grains if you want to lose weight, especially breads and pasta because they contain high levels of carrageenan and glutamate, which can harm your liver.

Make Smart Snacks if You Must

Although snacking is a common American past time, it should only be done in moderation to prevent intestinal injury and habituation. Walnuts and other nuts have anticancer properties due to their ellagic acid content, however allergies can result from excessive glutamate levels. Due to glutamate triggers, chocolate and nuts should be avoided by those who suffer from migraine headaches, while dark chocolate has heart and brain benefits.

Avert sweetened beverages and fruit juices.

Tea and fruit juices are high in sugar and might cause blood sugar levels to rise. It is best to use distilled water because black tea has fluoride and aluminum in it. Catechins, found in white and green teas, are beneficial to health and have anticancer properties. You can use monk fruit as a sweetener.

Test for Diabetes

According to recent studies, pre-diabetes is more common in Americans than diabetes, affecting one in four of them. Diabetes frequently has years without any symptoms; thus, screening is essential. The easiest method of screening for diabetes in the absence of symptoms is a urinalysis. Normal blood sugar levels are less than 100, however blood sugar levels above 100 need to be managed with diet and lifestyle modifications.

If you are over 45 and have one or more of the following risk factors, you should get tested for diabetes:

- A history of cardiovascular disease
- Are you inactive?
- Are overweight or obese
- Have a parent, brother, or sister with diabetes
- Have a family background that is African American, Alaska Native, American Indian, Asian American, Hispanic/Latino, or Pacific Islander

- Gave birth to a baby weighing more than 9 pounds or have been diagnosed with gestational diabetes, which is a temporary form of diabetes that occurs during pregnancy
- Have high blood pressure
- Have a triglyceride level above 250 mg/dL
- Have an elevated hs-CRP level
- Have polycystic ovary syndrome, also called PCOS
- Have other conditions associated with insulin resistance, such as a condition called acanthosis nigricans, characterized by a dark, velvety rash around the neck or armpits.

Control Blood Sugar: Natural Supplements

It has been discovered that certain natural substances lessen the consequences of both type 2 and type 1 diabetes, lowering blood sugar and inflammation. These substances have fewer negative effects and are safer. Additionally, they lessen the damage caused by lipid peroxidation and free radicals, which are the most detrimental mechanisms linked to diabetes. Damage to tissues and organs results from oxidative stress and inflammation brought on by impaired insulin action. Complications may arise from using drugs in excess or insufficiently. Advanced glycation end products (AGEs), which impair cell function, can result from untreated diabetes.

Using natural chemicals has the advantage of improving insulin action while also lowering inflammation, AGEs, and being potent antioxidants. Among the most successful are:

- Nano-Berberine
- R-lipoic acid
- Nano-Quercetin
- Nano-Curcumin
- Nano-Ginger extract
- Nano-Boswellia

CHAPTER 11

Fatty Liver illness

Often referred to as the "silent" liver disease, this illness is becoming more prevalent and has supplanted excessive alcohol use as the leading cause of liver disease. It is now the main reason liver transplants are performed in the United States. The primary risk associated with fatty liver disease is that, in its early stages, it rarely manifests any symptoms until the liver is seriously damaged, at which point the damage may already be severe.

Nonalcoholic fatty liver disease (NAFLD) and nonalcoholic steatohepatitis (NASH) are the two types of fatty liver disease. Overweight fat cells in the liver are the hallmark of nonalcoholic fatty liver disease (NAFLD), which affects 10–20% of Americans. Conversely, NASH damages the liver and induces inflammation, which results in cirrhosis and liver fibrosis. Although 3-26% of instances with NAFLD might result in significant damage and require a liver transplant, the condition can remain stable for years. Although it is uncommon, NASH is also connected to liver cancer. By concentrating on NASH and other causes of liver inflammation, the cure rate for hepatitis C has increased to 95%. Diet, exercise, weight loss, and refraining from needless medication are examples of current therapy. The only treatment available if the illness worsens and results in liver failure is a liver transplant.

Symptoms of Fatty Liver Disease

Since fatty liver disease usually shows no symptoms, it is referred to as a "silent killer". When it occurs, the symptoms—such as weariness, weakness, or discomfort in the abdomen—are typically ignored or misdiagnosed as other illnesses. Even if the illness develops into NASH, there could not be any signs until the When aberrant fat in the liver is combined with inflammation and liver damage, the symptoms usually go away quickly, but they can include fatigue, weakness, abdominal pain in the right upper quadrant, and weight loss. Similar to cirrhosis, significant liver hardness and scarring obstructs normal liver function, leading to the following symptoms:

- Swollen belly (fluid retention)
- Yellowish skin and eyes (jaundice)
- Intestinal bleeding
- Muscle wasting
- Liver cancer
- Liver failure liver damage becomes serious.

Risk Factors for NAFLD and NASH

Obesity

The main cause of non-alcoholic fatty liver disease (NAFLD), which is becoming more common, especially in young people, is obesity. The risk of developing fatty liver disease is seven to ten times higher in obesity. The rise in foods high in fructose corn syrup and foods containing excitotoxins is the main cause of the obesity pandemic. One of the main causes of chronic illnesses like NAFLD is persistent bodily inflammation, which is brought on by obesity. While there is no test that can identify which NAFLD patients will go on to develop NASH, there are risk factors that raise the possibility.

Gender

Although studies indicates that women may potentially be at higher risk after menopause, males have historically been at higher risk for NAFLD and NASH. This was discovered in a 2020 review of 60 papers for both NAFLD and NASH; however, the risk was minimal for women who had normal blood sugar, insulin, and weight.

Heredity

Although NASH can run in families, there is a type of the illness that is not absolutely hereditary. If either your father's or mother's side of the family has a history of NASH, discuss this with your physician. Your genetic susceptibility to NASH may be hereditary, therefore being overweight may not matter. It is also crucial to remember that abdominal obesity—which can occasionally affect skinny individuals—is the biggest cause of NASH.

Diabetes

A risk factor for non-alcoholic fatty liver disease (NAFLD) is insulin resistance or type 2 diabetes, which is the most prevalent type of the disease. This is because an excess of free fatty acids builds up in the bloodstream as a result of improper insulin response in the muscle, liver, and fat cells. Certain fat molecules have the potential to accumulate in the liver and cause harm due to inflammation. Fat cells accumulate more fatty acids when there is inflammation.

Metabolic Syndrome

This phrase describes a group of circumstances that raise the likelihood of fatty liver disease, including the likelihood of developing NASH, considerably. If a person has three or more of the following disorders, their condition is known as metabolic syndrome: high blood pressure, insulin resistance, glucose intolerance, high triglycerides, and abdominal obesity. Inflammation is another consequence of metabolic syndrome and is thought to have a major role in NASH and fatty liver disease.

Diabetes type 2 is closely associated with metabolic syndrome.

The Heart-Damaging Effects of Fatty Liver Disease

Regardless of the type of fatty liver disease you have, you should be concerned about the effects it may have on your heart because cardiovascular disease, which includes heart attacks and strokes, is the most prevalent cause of death for those with this condition. A small percentage of patients with fatty liver disease are afflicted by NASH, despite the fact that it can be fatal. Cardiovascular and cerebrovascular diseases, which include heart attacks and strokes (cerebrovascular disease), are the leading causes of death for those with fatty liver disease. Patients with fatty liver disease should be closely watched by their healthcare providers since they have an increased risk of having the following heart issues. Among these prerequisites are:

- **Coronary heart disease:** the coronary artery narrowing in the heart, which prepares the body for a heart attack. A stroke may result from this happening in the blood arteries supplying the brain.

- **Left ventricular hypertrophy:** An independent predictor of coronary heart disease, sudden death, heart failure, and stroke is an expansion and weakness of the heart's main pumping chamber.

- **Increased fat within the heart:** This aging-related syndrome is a sign of severe coronary heart disease. This condition is frequently disregarded.

- **Damage to the heart valves:** such include calcification of the mitral valve and aortic stenosis, both of which impair heart function.

- **Cardiac arrhythmias:** Heart attacks can result from electrical conduction problems, such as heart blockages of different degrees, and cardiac rhythms, such as atrial fibrillation and ventricular fibrillation.

The Cure for Fatty Liver Disease

Nonalcoholic fatty liver disease cannot currently be cured medically, but it can be avoided or, in some cases, even reversed if detected early. Here's how to carry it out:

- **Lose weight:** You can lower your risk by losing even 10% of your body weight.
- **Exercise daily:** For instance, a 2020 study showed that aerobic exercise helped individuals with non-alcoholic fatty liver disease. Every kind of exercise is beneficial.
- **Eliminate all foods containing sugar:** It comprises cake, pies, and candies in addition to other sugars that are "hidden" and present in packaged and processed foods. Instead, go for whole foods that are organic.
- **Avoid artificial sweeteners:** in particular, Splenda, saccharin, and aspartame.

- **Eliminate fried foods:** any dish prepared or cooked with omega-6 fatty acids.

- **Eliminate MSG:** and all food additives that include excitotoxins (natural flavors, hydrolyzed proteins, isolates or extracts of soy protein, autolyzed yeast, carrageenan, broth, etc.).

- **Cut out foods containing high-fructose corn syrup:** This, since it turns into fat more quickly and increases inflammation, may be contributing to the epidemic of fatty liver disease. (Refer to the prior suggestions.)

- **Eat lots of steamed cruciferous veggies:** According to recent studies, indole-3 carbinol, a naturally occurring substance present in a wide variety of plants, may reduce liver fat and inflammation. Brussels sprouts, cauliflower, kale, and cabbage are examples of cruciferous vegetables.

- **Avoid all unnecessary medications:** that, when feasible, put the liver under stress (label warnings should specify this).

- **Avoid all sources of fluoride:** found in black tea, public drinking water, raisins, and other dried fruits. To get rid of fluoride from your water, use a filter or sip distilled water.

- **Dietary fats do not directly cause liver disease:** However, because they exacerbate inflammation in the liver and all other tissues and organs, omega6 oils—such as those found in corn, safflower, sunflower, peanut, and soybean oils—should be avoided.

- **Drink white or green teas:** According to a number of studies, the catechin in these not only helps with weight loss but also lowers inflammation and other possible liver fat-reducing elements.

CHAPTER 12

The Liver Cirrhosis

A disease known as cirrhosis affects the liver and can cause variceal bleeding, ascites, spontaneous bacterial peritonitis, and hepatic encephalopathy, among other problems. Although it does not usually occur in illnesses that damage the liver, it is the most hazardous nonmalignant process affecting the liver. Nonalcoholic fatty liver disorders (NAFLD) and viral hepatitis, particularly those caused by type C and B hepatitis viruses, are associated with a higher incidence of cirrhosis. Liver fibrosis, in which collagen accumulates in the lobules of the liver, is the initial stage of liver injury. The hepatic portal system, the liver's blood drainage system, is hampered by processes that result in dense fibrous bands, regenerating nodules, and other liver function impairments. Hemorrhoids and ascites are brought on by an accumulation of fluid in the abdomen when this system is obstructed. Blocking the veins surrounding the lower esophagus can cause severe bleeding into the stomach and esophagus, which can worsen kidney function and perhaps cause death quickly.

The most prevalent kind of advanced chronic liver disease is cirrhosis, which, depending on the underlying cause, might take decades to fully develop. Compared to chemical damage, such as exposure to carbon tetrachloride, chronic viral liver damage can take longer to progress to cirrhosis. In the United States, 1% of people have cirrhosis, yet many cases go undiagnosed until an autopsy or routine laboratory test is performed. The development of cirrhosis may also be influenced by preexisting liver injury. Hepatitis B is the most common cause in Asia and sub-Saharan regions, but alcoholic liver disease and the hepatitis C virus are the most common causes in the West. In the United States, cirrhosis was linked to 25,000 fatalities and 373,000 hospital admissions in 1998.

Major Causes of Cirrhosis

Hepatitis C

The most frequent cause of cirrhosis is hepatitis C, which marginally surpasses persistent alcohol misuse. Hepatitis C is the far more common cause of cirrhosis, while hepatitis B and D can also cause it.

Chronic Alcohol Abuse

Heavy drinking—defined as consuming five or more drinks in a single day on at least five of the preceding thirty days—causes cirrhosis, a liver ailment. According to a 2008 study, moderate alcohol use raises the risk of cirrhosis, particularly in those who drink on a daily or non-mealtime basis. The risk of alcohol-induced cirrhosis is also markedly increased by the regular use of other liver toxic substances, exposure to industrial toxins, pesticides, herbicides, and some prescription medicines.

Nonalcoholic Fatty Liver Disease (NAFLD)

It is a very rare cause of cirrhosis because most of these cases do not lead to significant liver damage. When such cases are connected to the development of NASH and liver fibrosis, other factors like alcohol abuse, obesity, undiagnosed viral hepatitis, exposure to toxic chemicals that affect the liver, and advanced age, particularly in elderly patients who are weak, are usually implicated. For healthy elders, the risk is negligible even at the oldest ages.

Lesser Cirrhosis Causes

- Iron buildup in the body (hemochromatosis))
- Cystic fibrosis
- Copper was accumulated in the liver (Wilson's disease)
- biliary atresia, or inadequately formed bile tubes)
- Alpha-1 antitrypsin deficiency

- Genetic disorders that impact the way sugar is metabolized, such as glycogen storage disease and galactosemia
- genetically based intestinal disease (Alagille syndrome)
- liver disease associated with the immune system (autoimmune hepatitis)
- damage to the bile ducts (primary biliary cirrhosis)
- bile duct hardening and scarring (primary sclerosing cholangitis)
- An infection, such brucellosis or syphilis
- drugs, such as isoniazid or methotrexate.

Risk Factors for Different Types of Cirrhosis

Excessive Alcohol Consumption

There is a misconception that excessive drinking causes cirrhosis in all cases. Although alcohol misuse is a significant contributor to cirrhosis, there are other conditions that can also result in this type of liver damage. Contrary to popular belief, not everyone who drinks a lot gets cirrhosis; some people simply have livers that are more susceptible to the effects of alcohol. The majority of these cases involve drug addiction or an unhealthy diet. If alcohol consumption persists after liver disease has been identified, the liver will decompose much more quickly, which will result in severe cirrhosis. Over a five-year period, mortality increases to 85% after hepatic decompensation. Because alcohol is an immunosuppressive substance, quitting it can often worsen liver function by triggering an overreaction of the liver's immune system, which can lead to more damage. Steroids are used to manage this. Numerous natural remedies can lessen hepatic damage and stop an autoimmune response. This comprises nano-curcumin, nano-quercetin, nano-silymarin, and vitamin D3.

Obesity

Being overweight or obese raises your risk of nonalcoholic steatohepatitis (NASH) and nonalcoholic fatty liver disease (NAFLD), two diseases that can cause cirrhosis. Because obesity increases chronic inflammation, it is strongly linked to insulin resistance, type 2 diabetes, and the metabolic syndrome. Because obesity is associated with chronic inflammation, it is also highly associated with pancreatic cancer and hepatocellular carcinoma of the liver, two extremely lethal malignancies with a 4–8% five-year survival rate. Actually, having an infection with hepatitis B or C is not as significant of a risk factor for hepatocellular carcinoma as obesity is. The high prevalence of type 2 diabetes, which is likewise highly associated with the risk of hepatocellular carcinoma, is another factor linking obesity. The chance of acquiring these cancers increases significantly when drinking, smoking, and the use of oral contraceptives are combined with obesity.

Viral Hepatitis

Although cirrhosis is not a common outcome of chronic hepatitis, it is a risk factor. As was previously mentioned, a poor diet, exposure to pesticides, herbicides, or industrial chemicals, alcohol consumption, aspartame use, NAFLD, diabetes, obesity, and diabetes are just a few of the conditions that can exacerbate the negative effects of viral hepatitis or any other cause of liver damage.

Cirrhosis and Gender

In general, cirrhosis kills twice as many men as it does women. But women are additionally vulnerable because their stomachs lack the enzymes necessary to properly break down alcohol. As a result, the liver will get more alcohol and develop scar tissue.

Cirrhosis and Age

Most people believe that those who are older have a higher risk of developing cirrhosis. However, the onset of alcoholic cirrhosis symptoms can occur in people between the ages of 30 and 40, and they may not show up until the illness worsens. Alcoholic cirrhosis is also occurring in people at younger ages. According to a study that monitored cirrhosis-related deaths over a ten-year period, deaths in the 25–34 age range increased by 65%, with alcohol-related deaths accounting for the majority of the rise. Individuals who are older may be more susceptible to liver injury due to a decrease in the effectiveness of detoxifying enzymes, protective antioxidant enzymes, and glutathione. An appropriate diet, along with the application of specific nutritional supplements and flavonoids, can greatly improve liver function in older adults.

Symptoms of Cirrhosis

Some patients never have any symptoms at all, and their condition only shows up when their liver is severely damaged. The following indications could manifest earlier:

- feeling exhausted or weak
- easily cut or bruised
- Losing weight without exercising decreasing appetite vomiting and sickness
- little pain or suffering
- Edema, or ankle, foot, or leg swelling
- Skin irritation
- Jaundice is a yellow coloring of the skin and eyes. Ascites is a buildup of fluid in the belly.

- Spider-like skin blood vessels
- Redness on the hands' palms
- Absence of periods or total absence of them in women, unrelated to menopause
- Testicular atrophy, gynecomastia (enlarged breasts), or loss of libido drive
- speech slurred, tired, and confused (early hepatic encephalopathy).

Liver cirrhosis can result in ascites, bacterial peritonitis, bleeding from the stomach and esophagus, a rise in bacterial infections, and generalized inflammation. Hepatic encephalopathy can worsen until it puts the patient in a coma and eventually results in death. In 16–20% of patients with ascites, hepatopulmonary syndrome—a disorder characterized by an excess of nitric oxide produced in the pulmonary arteries—can result in hypoxemia and Porto pulmonary hypertension. These symptoms call for immediate medical attention since they show a fast decline in liver function. Cirrhosis was once thought to be a progressive illness requiring a liver transplant. Recent research indicates that a number of therapies can stop this process and restore the liver's natural functions. Researchers discovered that in 75 of the 153 cirrhosis cases with biopsy evidence, damage reversal happened following therapy of the underlying causes. More than any other organ in the body, the liver can renew itself. It has been shown that certain natural substances can shield the liver from harm and either halt or reverse the course of liver disease.

Diagnosis

The following tests are typically performed in order to diagnose cirrhosis:

Laboratory Tests

Transaminases, or liver enzymes, are among the first markers of liver disease when they are high. However, liver enzyme levels can remain normal or very slightly elevated for extended periods of time in cirrhosis patients. A test known as the international normalized ratio (INR) will be performed to see whether your blood is clotting normally because the liver is important for blood clotting. Serum albumin is another test used to assess the liver's capacity to synthesis this vital blood protein.

Imaging Tests

Although MRIs, CT scans, and ultrasounds may not be sensitive enough to fully diagnose cirrhosis, they can raise additional doubts about its presence. The characteristic expansion (hypertrophy) of the left liver lobe and shrinkage (atrophy) of the right liver lobe may be seen on the ultrasonography. A helical MRI with contrast can identify liver cancer or vascular disorders of the liver, but the MRI and CT scans are unable to determine the extent of the cirrhosis. An excess of iron in the liver, as observed in hemochromatosis, and an excess of fat in the liver linked to fatty liver illnesses (NAFLD and NASH) can both be detected by an MRI scan. It might be advised to use magnetic resonance elastography (MRE). The liver's elasticity, which is diminished with severe cirrhosis, is measured by the Fibro Scan. Pulse ultrasonography is used in the Shear Wave test to identify liver fibrosis. The fact that these tests don't involve surgery or needle biopsies is an advantage.

Biopsy

Since a liver biopsy makes it possible to directly determine the level of histologic damage and the degree of fibrosis, it is regarded as the gold standard for diagnosis. There are four stages of cirrhosis damage. A biopsy, or tissue sample, can be harmful and is not always necessary for a diagnosis. In two to three percent of patients, excessive bleeding during a biopsy is a sign of advanced cirrhosis, which is linked to coagulation issues. The majority of bleeding issues happen 24 hours after the biopsy. A biopsy may be recommended by your doctor in order to determine the kind, degree, and cause of liver disease.

Prognosis Determination

The MELD (Model for End Stage Liver Disease) system and the Child-Pugh-Turotte (CPT) classification are the two primary systems used by experts in liver problems to assess the prognosis of cirrhosis. Based on a one-year survival projection, the CPT method assigns patients to A, B, or C classes according to the likelihood that problems will arise. Class A has a one-year survival rate of 100%, Class B is at 80%, and Class C is at 45%. Regardless of the etiology, the MELD approach is more accurate and forecasts the best 3-month survival. The creatinine, bilirubin, and INR are used to calculate the score. It also determines which patients have a higher risk of passing away before receiving a liver transplant.

Hepatic Encephalopathy

Severe brain damage, from moderate to severe (coma), can result from liver destruction. Porto-systemic shunting procedures or cirrhosis may be the cause of this harm. Mental health disorders can also be brought on by other conditions such infections, renal failure, drug abuse, and previous neuropsychiatric disorders. There is a clear correlation between infections and brain impairment: 42% of patients without infections, 79% of patients with infections, and 90% of patients with severe infections (sepsis) all show signs of cognitive impairment. Based on the severity of the mental health issue, the West Haven Criteria assigns a class to mental function impairment.

Grade 1

- slight ignorance
- Either anxiety or euphoria
- little capacity for focus
- reduced capacity for addition and subtraction

Grade 2

- Apathy or lethargic behavior
- Changes in personality
- Time-displaced
- Unsuitable conduct

Grade 3

- Semi-stupor or somnolence
- Bewilderment Complete disorientation

Grade 4

- Regretfully, coma

Minimal hepatic encephalopathy concerns have gone unnoticed by the majority of doctors treating these individuals. The majority of the symptoms are thought to be modest, yet they can nonetheless negatively impact a person's quality of life. The following are possible experiences:

- Disturbances in sleep Falls
- Incompetent driving (repeated auto accidents)
- Issues related to work negatively impact survival

To identify mental impairment in liver cirrhosis, specialized tests such as the EEG, scan test, Clicker-Flicker frequency test (CFF), and psychometric hepatic encephalopathy test are utilized. Although the exact reason of declining brain function is unknown, there is compelling evidence that inflammation of the liver triggers the release of inflammatory chemicals and excitotoxins by immune cells known as microglia, which in turn harms brain tissue, particularly in the hippocampus region. Because infections cause a great deal of inflammation and activate brain microglia, this process is also connected to infections. The majority of experts blame excessive ammonium excreted from the intestines for the issue, but there may be more factors at play. According to studies, elevated ammonia levels by themselves have little effect and only become problematic when an infection is also present. Death is imminent as the encephalopathy deepens, but earlier stages—particularly the minimum stage—can be recovered from. Hepatic encephalopathy can also be improved by treatments like L-carnitine, which can improve mental performance and lower ammonia levels when taken in a quantity of two grams.

Treatment for Cirrhosis

Although cirrhosis cannot be cured, there are several things your doctor can do to control it and try to stop it from getting worse. Your prognosis will be determined by your general state of health and the existence of any cirrhosis-related problems. This remains valid even after abstaining from alcohol. First, your doctor will treat any underlying medical disorders that may be the cause of your cirrhosis, such as nonalcoholic fatty liver disease, chronic hepatitis B or C, or one of the less common reasons. Enrolling in an alcohol rehabilitation treatment program is essential if your cirrhosis is the result of alcohol addiction, as treatment cannot be advanced if a patient continues to consume alcohol.

Diet

People who have alcoholic cirrhosis should consume a well-balanced diet that mostly consists of organic meats and vegetables and moderately less salt. Increased consumption of branched chain amino acids (leucine, isoleucine, and valine) should also be a major component of the diet, as these acids have been shown to be helpful in cirrhosis of all kinds, not only alcoholic ones. The potential advantages of these nutrients were demonstrated by a man who underwent a three-week course of treatment with an amino acid mixture after suffering a severe alcoholic back surgery and not healing. In all cases of alcoholic cirrhosis, it is recommended to abstain from all alcohol, including wine.

Non-absorbable Disaccharides and Polyethylene Glycol

Many, but not all, investigations have demonstrated that the non-absorbed sugar substitute levulose improves hepatic encephalopathy. Compared to lactulose, polyethylene glycol appears to have a quicker symptom-reversal rate.

Antibiotics

It appears that non-absorbing antibiotics are more effective than absorbable ones. These antibiotics target bacteria in the colon and intestines, which can be a significant source of harmful substances like ammonia. Extensive research has demonstrated that the combination of lactulose and antibiotics was most effective in repairing the brain damage caused by cirrhosis.

Natural Products for Protecting and Treating Liver Diseases

Probiotics

According to a study, probiotics and prebiotics together help lessen hepatic encephalopathy. Probiotic-containing yogurt was administered to patients with cirrhosis and mild hepatic encephalopathy, while yogurt without probiotics was given to the control group. In cognitive tests, the probiotic yogurt significantly improved performance. On the other hand, neither the levels of inflammatory cytokines nor ammonia decreased. Lactose was secreted by all probiotic bacteria, and this could have fed damaged brain cells.

Zinc

Low blood and liver zinc levels are known to be linked to cirrhosis. Zinc, when combined with lactulose, considerably alleviated the neuropsychiatric symptoms, at least in moderate cases of hepatic encephalopathy, according to a study of four large trials involving 247 cirrhotic patients. Zinc picolinate, 50 mg per day, is a safe dosage.

Nano-Curcumin

Turmeric contains a chemical called curcumin, which has been shown to be beneficial in treating liver diseases, especially cirrhosis and fibrosis. The antiviral characteristics of this substance prevent the reproduction of multiple viruses, such as hepatitis B, hepatitis C, herpes simplex-1, influenza, human papillomavirus, and HIV. Additionally, curcumin lessens immunological damage to the liver and other organs and has a potent anti-transforming growth factor beta (TGF-ß1) effect. It raises glutathione levels, strengthens liver antioxidant enzymes, and facilitates better bile flow from the liver. Treatment with curcumin reduces oxidative stress, inhibits lipid peroxidation, reduces scar formation, and suppresses the production of inflammatory cytokines, so improving alcoholic liver damage dramatically. It also lessens the buildup of fat in the liver and is especially helpful in the treatment of non-alcoholic steatohepatitis (NASH), a more inflammatory fatty liver disease. 1000 mg of curcumin per day significantly improved quality-of-life metrics, such as physical and mental health ratings, in a trial including 70 cirrhosis patients. Curcumin is the most effective anticancer agent against a wide range of cancer types, including hepatocellular cancer. It also improves the efficacy of radiation therapy and traditional chemotherapy in treating tumors. Because of its excellent absorbability and widespread dispersion throughout the body, including the brain, it has a large margin of safety.

Nano-Quercetin

Many studies have been conducted on the potential benefits of quercetin, a natural supplement having antibacterial, anti-inflammatory, and antioxidant characteristics, in the treatment of liver problems. Researchers discovered that quercetin, when taken at a modest dose, not only averted much of the damage but also corrected a large amount of liver damage already produced by a potent liver toxin (carbon tetrachloride) in a study employing a rat model of chemically induced cirrhosis. According to the study, quercetin greatly improved the liver's histological appearance, decreased lipid peroxidation, decreased scarring, and brought nitric oxide levels back to normal. It's crucial to remember that excessive amounts of quercetin might have negative effects, so it's best to stick to moderate dosages. The recommended dosage of Nano-Quercetin is 250 mg each capsule, taken with food three to four times a day. Considering that it can drop blood sugar, it should always be taken with food. Additionally, quercetin has been demonstrated to be helpful in fatty liver disease cases, particularly in cases of nonalcoholic steatohepatitis (NASH), a more severe form of the condition than benign nonalcoholic fatty liver disease (NAFLD). Increased inflammation, elevated lipid peroxidation and free radical levels, and significant scarring are associated with NASH. If left untreated, nonalcoholic steatohepatitis (NASH) can lead to severe cirrhosis and an increased risk of liver hepatocellular cancer. Quercetin has been shown to reduce ethanol levels and lipid peroxidation, balance out imbalances in colon probiotics, and stop oxidative stress—which eventually destroys the liver—all of which work together to prevent liver damage. Additionally, it addresses insulin sensitivity issues, which are a significant contributing factor to the onset of fatty liver illnesses. It also raises the concentration of a unique bacteria known as Akkermansia muciniphila, which plays a significant role in avoiding obesity.

Nano-Silymarin

Silymarin, a naturally occurring substance derived from the milk thistle plant, has been extensively researched in relation to liver problems. The Nano-Silymarin product is well absorbed and efficiently penetrates the liver despite its limited absorption. While silymarin in its raw form has been the subject of most investigations, products with higher absorption rates have demonstrated superior benefits in protecting and treating liver damage. Although one study utilized baboons, the majority of animal investigations have used mice and rats. For 36 months, the baboons were given a diet heavy in ethanol-type alcohol, which caused liver cirrhosis. For a duration of one year and eighteen months, half of the baboons received silymarin, and every six months, their livers were assessed. The baboons had significant histological liver damage and increased liver enzymes; the researchers discovered. Silymarin, on the other hand, dramatically reduced the damaging molecule 4-hydroxynoneal (4-HNE), which is not neutralized by vitamin antioxidants, and the histological picture of individuals treated with it was markedly improved. Treatment is most successful when started early in the course of the disease when the damage is less severe and the liver's regenerative capacity is still high. Silymarin has a high margin of safety and tolerability. A recent review of silymarin used for liver diseases found that it significantly reduced deaths from cirrhosis, drug-induced liver damage, and diabetes-linked liver damage.

CHAPTER 13

Liver Tumors

Hepatocellular carcinoma is the primary cause of cancer-related fatalities globally, with liver cancer coming in second. Liver cancer is an uncommon but deadly illness in the United States. Until a person has a chronic liver illness, such as viral hepatitis, fatty liver disease, cirrhosis, severe fibrosis, alcoholism, smoking, exposure to liver toxins, or diabetes, primary liver cancer is not a serious danger. Rarely, these disorders can raise the risk of liver injury owing to genetic abnormalities.

What Is Liver Cancer?

An unchecked proliferation of aberrant cells within the body is the cause of liver cancer. Because cancer cells continue to proliferate unchecked, it is frequently described as a wound that never heals. Chronic, low-grade inflammation is what propels this process of cell proliferation. It can happen in tissues and organs that are inflamed all the time due to a variety of conditions such injury, infection, parasite infection, autoimmune disease, or chemical agent exposure. Hepatocellular carcinoma, intrahepatic cholangiocarcinoma, malignancies of the extrahepatic bile ducts, cancer involving the ampulla of Vater, and hepatoblastoma are among the various forms of liver cancer that start in the liver cells. Compared to primary liver cancer, metastatic cancer is more common, spreading from various sites to the liver. Metastatic colon cancer is one kind of spreading cancer that bears the name of the organ in which it first appeared.

Primary liver cancer is defined as a cancer that starts in the liver, but secondary liver cancer is defined as a metastatic cancer that spreads to the liver from another organ, such as the colon or pancreas. Hepatocellular carcinoma is the most prevalent kind of liver cancer, and it starts in the primary hepatocyte form of liver cell.

Who Gets Liver Cancer?

In the United States, liver cancer is a rare and frequently related illness that causes 42,230 new cases of diagnosis each year and accounts for over

30,000 fatalities. Since 1980, the incidence of liver cancer has tripled and is rising quickly. Liver cancer is the fifth most prevalent cause of cancer-related mortality in males, with a 70% greater chance of developing in men than in women. A fat-cell-secreted hormone that is more prevalent in women can lower the risk of malignant liver cells. The highest incidence of liver cancer in the United States is seen in Asian Americans and Pacific Islanders. A fat-cell-secreted hormone that is more prevalent in women can lower the risk of malignant liver cells. The highest incidence of liver cancer in the United States is seen in Asian Americans and Pacific Islanders.

Thirty to fifty percent of occurrences of hepatocellular carcinoma are most commonly linked to chronic hepatitis C infection. Aflatoxin exposure, hereditary abnormalities, hepatitis B, cryptogenic cirrhosis, and alcohol misuse are other contributing factors. Individuals with advanced stages of liver fibrosis or cirrhosis, smoking, diabetes, multiple infections, high alcohol consumption, advanced liver fibrosis, liver toxic artificial sweeteners, and excitotoxic dietary additives are at the highest risk of developing liver cancer. When these cases are investigated further, a cause is typically found.

Liver Cancer, Obesity, and Metabolic Disorders

There is a high correlation between obesity and liver cancer among other types of cancer. A 16-year follow-up study including 900,000 participants revealed a robust correlation between obesity and many cancer forms, including liver cancer. Drinking alcohol elevated the risk of liver cancer from cryptogenic cirrhosis by an additional 11 times, while obesity increased the risk by three times. Many American individuals discovered that obese men had a 4.5-fold increased chance of dying from liver cancer when compared to guys of normal weight. Compared to people of normal weight, obese people with hepatitis C or B have a significantly increased chance of developing liver cancer. A higher risk of liver cancer also exists for obese individuals who use food additives containing excitotoxins, aspartame, or Splenda (sucralose). A person with type 2 diabetes has a 7.5-fold increased chance of developing liver cancer if they also have insulin resistance. Combining diabetes and obesity makes the disease worse; the risk of liver cancer increases 100 times in the affected individual. Fructose greatly raises the risk of liver cancer, particularly high-fructose corn syrup. According to a European study, 25% of individuals with nonalcoholic steatohepatitis (NASH) and 74% of obese patients had nonalcoholic fatty liver disease (NAFLD).

Fatty Liver Disease and the Risk of Liver Cancer

Rarely is NAFLD, a straightforward fatty liver disease devoid of inflammation, connected to liver cancer. On the other hand, liver cancer risk is much higher in those with NASH, a more severe inflammatory illness. This risk is further increased by several diseases that have been shown to exacerbate liver damage, including obesity, type 2 diabetes, exposure to drugs toxic to the liver, chronic viral hepatitis infection, smoking, alcohol consumption, and aging.

Fatty liver affects about 25–30% of Americans, and 25% of these people will progress to nonalcoholic steatohepatitis (NASH). Twenty-five percent of NASH patients will eventually get cirrhosis, which puts them at high risk of getting liver cancer. The primary reason for liver transplants is increasingly becoming linked to cirrhosis in NAFLD patients. Cirrhosis from hepatitis C is on the decline, but NASH doubles or triples the risk of liver cancer in people with chronic hepatitis C infection. On the other hand, hepatitis B infection and a fatty liver reduce the risk of liver cancer. Patients with metabolic problems such as type 2 diabetes, insulin resistance, or metabolic syndrome are typically older, female, and have both NAFLD and liver cancer.

Alcoholic Liver Disease and Liver Cancer

A major contributing factor to liver cirrhosis, which raises the possibility of liver cancer, is alcohol misuse. There is a linear correlation between daily alcohol use and the risk of liver cancer, according to a study including almost 10,000 participants. Drinkers who were moderately intoxicated did not significantly enhance their risk; however, three drinks or more did. The risk rose at 50 and 100 grams per day from 29 to 66%. There are other factors at play as well, including diets, genetics, exposure to other liver toxins, silent viral infections, protective nutritional supplements, and genetics. Drinking alcohol increases a person's risk of liver cancer by double in hepatitis C virus patients. Alcohol misuse is the most prevalent risk factor for liver cancer in the US and Italy. A ten-year period of 80 grams of alcohol use increases the risk five times. Although it is thought to take 23 years to abstain from alcohol, a study indicated that the risk decreases by 6 to 7% annually. Consuming vitamins and natural substances can aid in the healing of damaged liver tissue, lessen liver scarring, and stop liver cancer.

Categories of Liver Cancer

Liver tumors fall into two categories: benign tumors, which are usually benign, and liver malignancies, which are the more hazardous kind that spread. The hepatocellular carcinoma we have been talking about falls under the latter kind.

Benign Liver Tumors

Hepatic benign tumors are frequent. They often do not represent a significant risk to health and do not spread to other parts of the body. Benign liver tumors are really detected "incidentally," which means they are discovered if you have an MRI, CT scan, or ultrasound performed for a different ailment. This is because benign liver tumors typically do not present any symptoms. They hardly ever need medical attention. There are three types of benign liver tumors, which are as follows:

- **Hemangiomas:** Hemangiomas are the most prevalent kind of liver tumors; they are masses of aberrant blood vessels. Up to 5% of adults are thought to develop tiny hepatic hemangiomas. In women, they are more prevalent. These benign tumors typically don't cause any symptoms and don't require medical attention. In the event that symptoms do arise, either because of their location or magnitude, they can require surgical excision.

- **Focal nodular hyperplasia (FNHs):** These represent the second most prevalent type of benign hepatic tumors. These tumors don't hurt or need to be treated. These typically affect women in their 20s and 30s. In extremely rare circumstances, they might require surgical removal if they are huge or painful.

- **Hepatocellular adenomas:** These are less frequent benign liver tumors that mostly affect women who are fertile. Higher estrogen dosages from oral contraceptives have been connected to the development of these tumors. They don't usually cause issues. These can also affect women who take hormone supplements. Women in these situations are recommended to stop taking hormones or birth control tablets in order to stop their growth. Rarely, surgery can be required.

Metastatic Liver Cancer

Metastatic liver cancer is a dangerous condition that can migrate to other areas of the body and infiltrate and harm nearby tissues. Colorectal, renal cell carcinoma, melanomas, pancreatic, sarcomas, stomach, lung, and breast cancers are among the common cancer types to metastasize to the liver. About 50% of individuals with colorectal cancer experience liver metastases, making it the most prevalent form to do so. Slightly more than half of these tumors can be surgically eliminated. Approximately 40% of patients, according to recent studies, may live for five years following tumor removal; this is in contrast to less than 1% of patients who have multiple metastatic liver tumors.

For all tumor types, radiofrequency ablation and cryotherapy work marginally better and are less likely to propagate malignant cells.

Types of Primary Liver Cancers

Hepatocellular carcinoma: Three-quarters of all instances of liver cancer are hepatocarcinoma (HCC), also known as hepatoma. This is the most prevalent kind of liver cancer. It can spread to other areas of the body and begins in hepatocytes, which make up the majority of liver cells. HCC is more common in people with extensive liver disease, especially in those with cirrhosis, and it is most common in those who abuse alcohol. Less than 40% of HCC tumors are detected early in their development; most diagnoses occur later in the tumor's life. Despite standard treatment, the survival rate for patients with advanced HCC is low.

Cholangiocarcinoma: This less prevalent malignancy, also referred to as bile duct cancer, makes up as much as 20% of all liver cancer cases. Intrahepatic bile duct cancer is the name for cancer that starts inside the liver's bile ducts; extrahepatic bile duct cancer is the name for cancer that starts in the portion of the ducts outside the liver.

Liver angiosarcoma: Since this uncommon type of liver cancer tends to spread swiftly and starts in the liver's blood vessels, it is usually discovered at a later stage.

Hepatoblastoma: Almost always, this incredibly uncommon form of liver cancer is discovered in young children, typically younger than three.

Symptoms

Liver cancer is rarely diagnosed in its early stages, so by the time it manifests symptoms, it may have progressed. When they do, the following symptoms may appear:

- Abdominal discomfort, pain, and tenderness
- Jaundice
- White, chalky stools
- Nausea
- Vomiting
- Bruising or bleeding easily

- Weakness
- Fatigue

Is Liver Cancer Preventable?

According to research that was published in 2018 in CA: A Cancer Journal for Clinicians, a large number of instances are indeed preventable. This one study found that these avoidable causes account for 71% of liver cancer diagnoses in the United States. A higher risk of liver cancer is associated with:

- Hepatitis C, B, D, and HIV
- Excess body weight (obesity and overweight)
- Smoking
- Alcoholism
- Type 2 diabetes
- Metabolic syndrome
- Insulin resistance
- Nonalcoholic steatohepatitis–NASH (the severe form of fatty liver disease)
- Exposure to toxic liver compounds – Pesticides/herbicides – Industrial chemicals – Artificial sweeteners

(aspartame, sucralose, and saccharine) – Excitotoxic food additives (MSG, hydrolyzed proteins, soy protein extracts, etc.)

According to a study conducted by Farhad Islami, the American Cancer Society's strategy director for cancer surveillance research, avoiding risk factor exposure may be able to avert almost 50% of liver cancer fatalities. These hazards may be further decreased by using natural liver protectants such as apigenin, baicalin, berberine, nano-silymarin, nano-curcumin, and nano-quercetin.

Causes of Liver Cancer

- **Genetics:** Although hereditary hemochromatosis is not a hereditary condition, persons who have it may be more susceptible to liver cancer. This condition causes an excess of iron to be absorbed from diet. All around the body, tissues hold on to iron, but mostly in the liver. The accumulation of iron in the liver can cause cirrhosis and liver cancer. A higher risk of liver cancer is also associated with specific genetic markers, such as PNPLA3 and GTSM1. Wilson's illness is also linked to secondary liver cirrhosis caused by elevated tissue copper levels.

- **Existing liver disease:** People who have hemochromatosis in their family are more vulnerable, as said. Furthermore, Wilson's illness and hepatitis might develop into liver cancer. Hepatitis viruses can change the DNA of the liver by causing persistent, smoldering inflammation and increasing the liver's vulnerability to malignancy.

- **Alcohol use:** In the United States, alcohol misuse is a major contributor to cirrhosis, which is connected to a higher risk of liver cancer. Hepatocellular carcinoma and intrahepatic cholangiocarcinoma are the two forms of liver cancer that heavy drinkers are approximately twice as likely to develop.

- **Smoking:** Smokers who are currently in the habit have a 51–70% higher risk of developing liver cancer; even those who have stopped are still at danger, albeit somewhat. Research indicates that there is no additional risk for people who have stopped smoking for at least 30 years.

- **Type 2 diabetes:** Common forms of diabetes are associated with a higher risk of liver cancer, typically as a result of other conditions such chronic viral hepatitis and/or severe alcohol consumption. Additionally, type 2 diabetics frequently have obesity or excess weight, which can exacerbate liver issues.

- **Chemicals:** Certain chemical exposures can harm the liver. Chemicals that are used in the workplace include thorium dioxide (Thorotrast), a chemical that was once injected into patients as part of specific X-ray diagnostics, and vinyl chloride, which is used to create plastic. Thorotrast is no longer in use, and vinyl chloride is now strictly monitored. In addition to being a component of the vinyl chloride production process, arsenic is also present in drinking water and has been related to cancer risk and liver damage. Some liver cancer cases in Africa and other underdeveloped countries are caused by a chemical called aflatoxin, which is present in a particular kind of fungus. As previously reported, some aflatoxins can be found in some brand-name peanut butter.

- **Anabolic steroids:** Long-term usage of anabolic steroids, which are male hormones used by some sportsmen to gain more muscle mass and power, may slightly raise the chance of developing hepatocellular carcinoma. This risk is not associated with cortisone-like drugs, such as hydrocortisone, prednisone, and dexamethasone.

Diagnosing Liver Cancer

If detected early, liver cancer has a high 5-year survival rate of 33%; if it spreads to nearby tissues or organs, it has a rate of 11%; if it travels to distant portions of the body, it has a rate of 2%. While conventional treatments are employed, their effectiveness can be enhanced and negative effects mitigated when combined with plant extracts. Some people could choose to use natural remedies or a mix of them. However, because the liver is a big organ that develops symptoms slowly, liver cancer patients frequently remain undetected until the malignancy has progressed. A liver cancer screening is necessary if:

- You have a family history of liver cancer or cirrhosis.
- You have chronic hepatitis B or C.
- You have fatty liver disease.
- You have been exposed to known liver toxins.
- You drink more than three drinks a day every day.
- You are obese, especially if you have type 2 diabetes.
- You have hemochromatosis or Wilson's disease.

You should talk to your doctor about test screenings if you have any other risk factors for liver disease. Alpha-fetoprotein (AFP), a material that may be produced by cancer cells, can be detected in the blood as one of the screening alternatives.

Additionally, 20 to 25 percent of people with hepatitis, chronic cirrhosis, or other liver illnesses may have increased AFP. In other words, it is not exclusive to liver cancer. Non-invasive diagnostic tests including magnetic resonance imaging (MRI), computed tomography (CT) scans, and ultrasounds are examples of other diagnostic testing. The most accurate scan is an MRI, which also emits no radiation.

Liver Cancer Treatment

Hepatocellular carcinoma, the most prevalent type of liver cancer, has a number of possible treatments, especially when detected early. This type of liver cancer is often treated with one of two surgeries:

Surgery

The most effective disease-directed treatment for liver cancer is probably surgery, or partial hepatectomy, especially if your liver function is good and the tumors can be safely removed from a small area of your liver. If the patient has other significant conditions, the tumor has spread outside the liver, the liver is too damaged, or the tumor occupies too much space in the liver, surgery might not be an option. After this procedure, the malignant section of the liver is removed, and the remaining piece of the liver may grow back. A partial resection results in a 60% 5-year survival rate, compared to 70% with an early diagnosis. The 5-year tumor recurrence rate is 20–35% overall.

Liver Transplant

A donor liver replaces the damaged liver during a liver transplant, which involves the removal of the entire liver. Only certain conditions, such as the quantity and size of the tumors and the availability of a qualified donor, can make this surgery feasible. Because liver transplantation eliminates both the diseased liver and the tumor, it is a very successful treatment for patients with tiny tumors. But there aren't many donors, so you could have to wait a while for a liver to become available. There is a 15% risk of tumor recurrence in the replacement organ following liver transplantation.

Nonsurgical Treatments

Radiotherapy Ablation

Also referred to as thermal ablation, this minimally invasive procedure uses heat directed by a microwave through a tiny needle to eliminate the tumor. This therapy can be applied topically, via laparoscopy, or in conjunction with surgery.

Cryotherapy

In addition, a tiny probe is used percutaneously (through the skin) to freeze the tumor, killing it as well as preventing the tumor cells from spreading, which is a common occurrence with open surgery. Research has indicated that the act of freezing a tumor can trigger an immune response against any remaining tumor cells. The majority of treatment series yield better results than other approaches.

Stereotactic Body Radiation Therapy (SBRT)

With this procedure, substantial radiation doses are administered to the tumor while the radiation dosage to adjacent healthy tissue is kept to a minimum. carried out to treat tumors that are no larger than 5 cm.

Advanced Liver Cancer Treatments

For advanced liver cancer, the following therapies are taken into consideration:

Chemotherapy

Chemotherapy is the use of certain medications to kill cancer cells, usually by preventing the cancer cells from proliferating, dividing, or developing into new ones. In order to extend the period that the chemotherapy remains in the tumor, chemoembolization involves injecting medications into the hepatic artery, which is the blood vessel supplying the liver, temporarily obstructing the flow. These therapies have proven incredibly unsatisfactory and have major side effects.

Radioembolization

This process is comparable to chemoembolization, with the exception that radioactive beads are inserted into the artery supplying blood to the tumor.

When the beads get stuck in the tumor's tiny blood veins, they immediately begin to give radiation therapy to the tumor. The outcomes have not been that impressive.

Targeted Treatments

Drugs known as "targeted therapies" specifically target the genes, proteins, or tissue environment that the cancer uses to grow and survive. This kind of treatment lessens harm to healthy cells while preventing the growth and spread of malignant cells. They haven't really improved the course of treatment yet.

Immunotherapy

Immunotherapy, also known as biologic therapy, boosts the body's defenses against cancer by utilizing the immune system. An immune checkpoint inhibitor is a frequent form of immunotherapy. Immune checkpoint drugs function by obstructing the immune system-evading pathways that the malignancy would otherwise use to conceal itself. While there is likely a higher likelihood of success with these treatments, there is also a potential for serious, long-lasting negative effects.

CHAPTER 14

Transplanting Liver

Liver transplants have gained popularity as a treatment for acute and chronic illnesses leading to severe liver dysfunction during the last forty years. The organ that is transplanted most frequently is the liver, which is followed by the heart and lung. To replace the recipient's damaged liver, a complete or partial liver from a deceased or living donor is used in the process. The surgery is intricate and demands proper execution and cautious harvesting. Approximately 8000 liver transplants were carried out in the United States in 2017, of which 360 involved living donors. There were roughly 11,500 persons on the liver transplant waiting list.

How Successful Are Liver Transplants?

A liver transplant's likelihood of success depends on a number of variables, such as the surgeons' training and expertise and the transplant's intended use. Within the first year following the transplant, the majority of deaths happen in the first three months, frequently as a result of technical issues, initial graft failure, infection, and organ rejection. Chronic kidney failure, cancer, infections, chronic organ rejection and transplant failure, and cardiovascular disease are the main causes of mortality later in life. The majority of deaths that occur after a liver transplant are related to immunosuppressive disorders or side effects from the medications used to reduce rejection immunity.

The reason for the transplant, such as exposure to hazardous chemicals, viral hepatitis, alcoholic cirrhosis, or cryptogenic cirrhosis, will also determine the transplant's success. Ninety-five percent of patients with viral hepatitis receiving liver transplants will carry the virus in both their blood and the new liver. Less than half will, however, exhibit clinical symptoms of the infection, and within five years, 20 to 40 percent will develop cirrhosis of the new liver.

Compared to patients with end-stage liver disease from other causes, those with alcoholic cirrhosis have worse health, need more reoperations, and are younger. Resuming alcohol use after the transplant has a significant risk of damaging the newly transplanted liver in cases of alcoholic cirrhosis. Natural remedies that are known to shield the liver in similar circumstances help lessen these issues.

Seventy-five percent of liver transplant recipients live for at least five years on average; thirty die within five years, and 75 survive for five years. Perhaps because they are healthier than deceased donors, living donor recipients frequently have higher short-term survival rates than deceased donors.

Types of Liver Transplant

Deceased-Donor Transplants

When a deceased person donates their liver, doctors replace the damaged or diseased liver with the deceased donor's. This procedure is known as cadaveric donation. Although surgeons can divide the liver into smaller portions for smaller adults or toddlers, adults usually receive the full liver. Before being evaluated for transplantation, the liver is examined for viruses and compatibility. Since the organ's viability is limited, a speedy transplant is necessary to provide the best potential result. The liver transplant needs to be carried out as close to the donor as possible.

Living-Donor Liver Transplants

In a living-donor transplant, a family member who is in need of a liver transplant receives a portion of the liver of a healthy living individual. Although less prevalent, this treatment has benefits like greater health, a lower risk of problems, a higher chance of a successful transplant, shorter wait times, and the ability to know or be connected to the recipient. Surgeons remove a portion of the healthy liver of the donor during a living-donor transplant in order to replace the patient's damaged or diseased liver. Not long after the operation, the donor's liver returns to normal size, and the recipient's liver does too. Even though they are less frequent than transplants from deceased donors, living donors are becoming more and more common.

Domino Liver Transplants

A live donor with familial amyloidosis gives their liver to another living donor in a less usual procedure known as a "domino liver transplant." Internal organ damage and aberrant protein accumulation are the results of this rare illness. The receiver is eligible to receive the donor's liver since it is in good functioning order. Amyloidosis symptoms can appear at any time; however, they typically take decades to manifest. It is not anticipated that recipients, who are usually 55 years of age or older, will experience symptoms before the end of their natural lives.

Who Is Eligible for a Liver Transplant?

Typically, individuals with advanced liver disease fall into one of two categories. There are two types of situations: emergency cases, which require rapid evaluation for transplantation, and chronic cases, which steadily worsen liver function. These are the individuals that require liver transplants the most frequently. Individuals who have been under a doctor's care for a long time and have a chronic illness that is becoming worse are most frequently referred for liver transplants. This category includes several of the illnesses that were previously covered in this book, such as:

- Fatty liver disease (nonalcoholic steatohepatitis)
- Chronic viral hepatitis B and C
- Alcoholic liver disease
- Some types of liver cancer
- Certain autoimmune and genetic diseases
- Vascular diseases of the liver

A liver transplant may be required in cases of acute liver illness, which is frequently brought on by poisoning, overdosing, or blood channel blockage. But most people who have a history of active drug usage, a six-month alcohol abstinence period, or an organ illness like severe heart disease are not candidates for a liver transplant because they now use drugs or alcohol that could harm the new liver. Furthermore, people who suffer from advanced heart disease or other organ diseases might not be able to handle the stress of a transplant operation.

Disparities by Gender in Liver Transplants

There is a gender difference in liver transplantation, according to a review published in the Journal of Hepatology, with males obtaining the procedure more frequently, experiencing shorter waiting times, and having better results. The distinction is most noticeable in transplants brought on by hepatitis C. Most transplants happen to people between the ages of 50 and 64. Within three years of being added to a waiting list, women have a 30% lower chance of receiving a transplant, and they have a 9% lower chance of receiving transplants from living donors. In addition, women are more prone to experience disease or death. In order to comprehend the causes of this discrepancy, more investigation is required.

The Liver Transplant Center

Patients are referred to a specialized liver transplant clinic for additional assessment when their liver disease is no longer curable. Within the transplant center, the Liver Transplant Program is a multidisciplinary practice run by physicians, surgeons, and other specialists. There are more than 100 liver transplant centers in the United States, some of which are connected to university medical schools. In addition to their social support system, patients' physical, mental, and financial circumstances are taken into consideration when evaluating them. To ascertain the severity of the liver illness, liver function, and general body functioning, numerous medical tests are performed. Additionally, the team assesses whether there are any additional treatments that could prevent premature liver transplants. In cases where alcohol is a factor, referrals to counseling or rehabilitation programs can be required.

The following details are important to know while looking into a liver transplant center:

- Whether the center is located close to where you live.
- What is the annual count of liver transplants performed and what is the rate of patient survival? Large volume centers typically

have higher success rates because experience matters. This isn't always the case because the caliber of the surgeon matters more than the volume of transplants performed. A surgeon who performs many poor transplants is not as valuable as one who performs fewer effectively.

- How much it costs, if your health insurance will pay for it, and whether you have to make any copayments. This covers expenses incurred before to, during, and following the transplant as well as travel expenses and lodging costs (if any) if you need to stay close to the facility throughout your recuperation.
- Whether the center stays current with advancements in transplant science, technology, and methodology.

Benefits and Risks of Liver Transplantation

While there are many advantages to having a liver transplant, such as increased quality of life and survival rates, there are also risks. These include the need to take immunosuppressive medications for the rest of one's life in order to prevent the liver from being rejected, surgical complications, and the potential for recurrent liver disease. However, because the liver is such a vital organ to your health, by the time liver disease is severe, the advantages of a liver transplant typically exceed the risks.

Risks of Liver Transplantation

- Bile duct complications, including bile duct leaks or shrinking of the bile ducts
- Bleeding
- Blood clots
- Failure of the donated liver
- Infection
- Rejection of the donated liver
- Mental confusion or seizures

Risks of Anti-rejection Drugs

- Bone thinning
- Diabetes
- Diarrhea
- Headaches
- High blood pressure
- High cholesterol

Waiting for a Liver Transplant

As of 2017, the waiting list for a liver transplant from a dead donor was 239 days long. Potential recipients of a liver transplant are added to a nationwide database maintained by the United Network for Organ Sharing (UNOS), which offers details about the procedure. In order to enhance the procedure of matching intestine and liver organs to candidates who have the greatest need, the Organ Procurement and Transplantation Network (OPTN) was established in 2019. Eleven transplant zones and fifty-eight donor service areas (DSAs) were used as geographic borders before the current system was implemented. The Model for End-Stage Liver Disease (MELD), created by UNOS to assess the severity of the condition in patients awaiting liver transplantation, serves as the foundation for the ultimate determination. The most critically sick individuals have the highest MELD scores, which range from 6 to 40. When allocating organs, race, sex, or ethnic background are irrelevant considerations. The availability of organs, the patient's blood type, and the medical urgency indicated by their MELD score all affect a person's place on the waiting list. For the majority of patients with chronic liver disease, the MELD score can predict the risk of death or the 3-month and 1-year mortality. Decisions on transplantation must be taken within a few days in extremely urgent circumstances.

Liver Transplant Procedure

A sick donor's liver is surgically removed and transplanted into the body of the recipient during a liver transplant operation. A medical examination is conducted to make sure the recipient is healthy enough for the general anesthetic operation. The liver is accessed by the surgeon through a lengthy incision across the abdomen. The damaged liver is removed, and the donor liver's blood arteries and bile ducts are connected. The incision is closed by the surgeon using staples and stitches when the new liver is positioned. After that, the patient is brought to the intensive care unit so they can heal. The surgery is planned ahead of time if the donor is a living person. Both the donor's and the transplanted livers regenerate quickly, returning to normal volume in a matter of weeks. After a liver transplant, recovery usually lasts three to six months.

After a Liver Transplant

You will need to take every necessary step to maintain the health of your newly transplanted liver. The National Institute of Diabetes and Digestive and Kidney Diseases has the following recommendations:

- Take medicines exactly as your doctor tells you to take them.
- Before taking any additional medications, including over-the-counter and prescription drugs, vitamins, and nutritional supplements, with your doctor.

- Don't miss any scheduled blood draws or medical visits.
- Stay away from people who are sick.
- Tell your doctor when you are sick.
- Learn to recognize the symptoms of rejection.
- Have cancer screenings as recommended by your doctor.
- Consult your physician about the use of birth control and the possible risks and consequences of becoming pregnant, both before and after your liver transplant.

Diet and Liver Transplantation

The two main causes of liver transplant failure are immunological rejection and infection. In a rat research, rats given a diet rich in omega-3 oils had a 100% survival rate within 30 hours post-surgery, and 20% of the rats receiving the oil were still alive two weeks later. The rats on special diets demonstrated notable liver regeneration and the restoration of the unique architecture of the liver. Additionally, they exhibited increased concentrations of IL-4 and IL-10, two cytokines that lower immunological rejection and liver inflammation and may help avoid liver rejection.

According to a study, patients receiving liver transplants for end-stage liver disease or liver cancer who also took omega-3 oil had much lower liver enzyme levels, less damage to their liver cells, shorter hospital stays, and fewer issues overall—particularly postoperative infections. When comparing those on the omega-3 diet to those on the normal diet, three times as many persons died.

The DHA type of omega-3 oils, particularly the triglyceride formulation, is the safest and most effective form available. DHA is provided in the triglyceride form in the Garden of Life DHA supplement, with a daily dose of 1000–2000 mg. DHA increases the tolerance and longevity of donated organs, according to studies.

Through the regulation of immune cell receptors and the inhibition of inflammation in the liver through a variety of methods, curcumin has been demonstrated to block the major inflammatory pathways that are triggered during transplanted liver rejection. But before utilizing any compound, it's crucial to speak with a doctor.

CHAPTER 15

What to Eat for a Healthy Liver?

Sustaining general body homeostasis requires keeping a healthy liver. A healthy diet is vital for the liver, which is in charge of metabolizing food and liquids. Proteins, lipids, and carbohydrates that are absorbed by the digestive system enter the bloodstream and are subsequently metabolized by the liver. Additionally, the liver prevents dangerous drugs like alcohol from building up in the body by neutralizing them. As a result, preserving general bodily balance and guaranteeing the efficient execution of bodily processes depend on a healthy liver.

Eating for a Healthy or Healing Liver

What to Avoid:

- Foods's high in fat, sugar, and salt
- Fried foods
- raw or undercooked shellfish, such as oysters and clams; oysters feed by filtering

surrounding water where waterborne bacteria (vibrio) may thrive, possibly leading to the bacteria multiplying in the human body and causing disease. Omega-6 fats are found in margarine, salad dressings, cooking oils, and added to most processed foods.

- **Alcohol:** You might need to give up alcohol completely if you have liver disease, depending on the sort of liver disease you have. If not, limit your daily alcohol intake to one drink for women and two for men.

Eat a Balanced Diet

Choose from a variety of nutritious food groups, including fruits, vegetables, lean meats, legumes, and healthy oils like coconut and extra virgin olive oil. The taste of coconut bothers some people. Thankfully, a refined version exists that doesn't taste or smell like coconut.

Eat Food with Fiber

Fiber supports the best possible function of your liver. Oatmeal, fruits, vegetables, and legumes help provide your body's fiber requirements.

Drink White or Green Tea and Adequate Amounts of Water

Drinking fluids keeps you from being dehydrated, improves liver function, and gives your liver strong antioxidants.

Diets

I support three distinct dietary approaches because of their benefits to the liver. First, try my anti-inflammatory diet, which is great for anyone trying to avoid chronic illnesses, especially liver-related ones. Benefits to the liver have also been shown for the Mediterranean diet and the DASH diet.

Eat and Drink Vegetables

Consume six servings or more of vegetables each day. Nutrient-dense vegetables like broccoli, Brussels sprouts, cauliflower, cabbage, onions, leeks, whole tomatoes, collards, mustard greens, spinach, kale, and celery should be a part of these servings.

Consume the Proper Proteins

Contrary to what your doctor may tell you, saturated fats have very little to do with cholesterol or heart disease. But, the fats from meats farmed organically are far safer than those from meats raised traditionally, which have smaller amounts of healthy fats and higher concentrations of industrial chemicals, pesticides, herbicides, and harmful metals. The ideal diet would consist of no more than 6 ounces of organic chicken, turkey, fish, and occasionally pork (unless your religion forbids it). You might also incorporate beef that has been fed on grass once or twice a week. I think of fish as a dietary group that includes meat, and I suggest consuming fish that has a high omega-3 fat content and a low mercury content. On both counts, wild salmon is an excellent option. Fish with varying mercury levels fluctuate over time.

Know Your Fats

Omega-6 oils, which are utilized as cooking oils, in salad dressings, and in the majority of processed foods, are unhealthy, inflammatory fats. They should be avoided and include canola, peanut, soybean, sunflower, corn, and safflower oils. These oils break down quickly due to oxidation, much like margarine does when it is left out of the refrigerator. They cause severe inflammation throughout the body, including in blood vessels. They are also known to promote the invasion, growth, and metastasis of cancer. Because many processed goods utilize a variety of these oils, carefully read the labels. While typical Western diets contain up to 50 times the required quantity of omega-6 fats, some of them are still necessary. You can obtain all the omega-6 fats you need from vegetables and organically reared animals, and in a far healthier form than from processed foods. Meat from calves raised on grass has more of the beneficial omega-3 oils. Extra virgin coconut oil is the best oil for cooking. Use refined coconut oil, which has no taste or odor, if you don't like the taste of coconut. Make use of extra virgin olive oil for salad dressings. Remember to read labels carefully. The claim in big letters on a lot of commercial products is that the dressing comprises "extra virgin olive oil," but in reality, it also contains a combination of omega-6 oils.

Healthy Drinks

The ideal drinks are white or green tea and purified water. Water purifies and hydrates without posing any risks. One of the more significant circulatory systems that helps the body get clean is the lymphatic system, which depends on proper hydration to function. In addition to being hydrated, white and green teas have anti-inflammatory and antioxidant properties. Select decaffeinated versions if you find that caffeine keeps you up at night or if you are sensitive to it. Fruit juices include a lot of sugar, fluoride, and sometimes metal, so I don't suggest them.

Avoid Trans Fats

Even when a label state there are no trans fats, these oils—which are listed as "partially hydrogenated" oils—can be found in a lot of processed goods. This is because if trans-fat content is less than 0.5 grams per serving, food standards permit a "zero" label. Even so, eating multiple portions of foods that contain almost half a gram per serving can quickly accumulate to harmful levels because simply a few grams of them per day can damage arteries. Checking to check if any partially hydrogenated oil is stated as an ingredient is the easiest approach to determine if the meal actually contains trans-fat. Recall that the liver is severely harmed when trans fats and MSG are combined.

Avoid Sugar

Sugar consumption is the most powerful association with heart attacks, strokes, and atherosclerosis rather than cholesterol or even lipids. All sugar-containing items (cakes, pies, candies, sweetened beverages, fruit juices, and other sources of sugar) should be eliminated, unless there are exceptional circumstances. Since high-fructose corn syrup is the worst, it should be steered clear of at all costs. Carefully read ingredient labels as this type of sugar can be included in many sauces, soups, and other foods that we wouldn't often identify with sugar in addition to plainly sweet items. Fruits should only be eaten in moderation due to their high sugar content. Best are fruit powders that have had most of the sugar removed.

Reduce Starchy Carbohydrates

Certain carbohydrates function in the human body similarly to sugar. Technically speaking, foods high in specific starches are referred to as "high-glycemic" carbs because, after consumption, they quickly turn into blood sugar. These consist of white or whole grain breads, buns, biscuits, rolls, chips, cereals, potatoes, and crackers. It's important to consider the "glycemic load," or the quantity of a specific starchy item you're consuming. A modest sum might work perfectly well.

Avoid Fluoride

This covers mouthwash, toothpaste, raisons, and other dry fruit in addition to black tea and fluoridated water. Due to its high reactivity, fluoride can harm tissues, cells, and organs even at very low quantities. This is particularly valid for kids. Fluoride is particularly harmful because it builds up in specific bodily tissues.

The DASH Diet

Dietary Approaches to Stop Hypertension, or DASH, is a long-term, health-oriented approach to eating well that aims to prevent or treat hypertension (high blood pressure), but it also has a host of other benefits, particularly for the liver.

What Kind of Diet Is DASH?

Here's a look at the recommended servings from each food group for the 2000-calories-a-day DASH diet. While the DASH diet is effective for controlling blood pressure, it contains many items I would not endorse for other reasons.

- **Grains: 6 to 8 Servings a Day:** Bread, cereal, rice, and pasta are examples of grains. One slice of whole-wheat bread, one ounce of dry cereal, or ½ cup of cooked cereal, rice, or pasta are a few examples of one serving of grains. I do not support eating grains, not on a regular basis. They contain high levels of the excitotoxin glutamate and lectins, both of which harm tissues. Most have a lot of gluten as well.

- **Vegetables: 4 to 5 Servings:** A Day Vegetables such as tomatoes, carrots, broccoli, sweet potatoes, and greens are rich in fiber, vitamins, and minerals including magnesium and potassium. One cup of raw leafy green vegetables or ½ cup of chopped raw or cooked veggies are examples of one serving. Glutamate and lectin levels are high in tomatoes. Particularly in tomato purees and sauces, glutamate is a cause for worry.

- **Fruits: 4 to 5 Servings a Day:** Similar to vegetables, fruits are generally low in fat and high in fiber, potassium, magnesium, and very healthy flavonoids (coconuts are an exception). Their sugar content is high (fructose). One medium fruit, ½ cup of fresh, frozen, or canned fruit, or four ounces of juice are examples of one serving. Ask your doctor or pharmacist if certain citrus fruits and juices, including grapefruit, are safe for you to consume. Certain drugs may interact with certain citrus fruits and drinks. Organic fruits should ideally be consumed whole rather than juiced; if the peels are edible, keep them on as they are a good source of fiber. Even fruits that are cultivated organically should be cleaned with a vegetable wash before consumption. Strawberries, blueberries, and raspberries are among of the healthiest fruits.

- **Dairy 2 to 3 Servings a Day:** Dairy products such as milk, yogurt, and cheese are excellent providers of protein, calcium, and vitamin D. Low-fat foods are better. The more recent DASH diet does not include this. Any sort of milk consumption should be avoided as it can promote the growth of cancer, particularly prostate cancer. The high calcium concentration is the reason of this. Cow's milk is likewise a high-allergen food and has relatively high glutamate levels. Never drink soy milk since it contains a lot of fluoride, aluminum, and glutamate and can harm your brain.

- **Lean Meat, Poultry, and Fish: Six 1-Ounce Servings, or Fewer, a Day:** Iron, zinc, B vitamins, and protein can all be found in abundance in meat. Limit your daily intake of meat to four or six 1-ounce portions, choosing from a variety of cuts. If desired, one can remove excess fat, although it's not necessary. Cooking oil should not be used while baking, broiling, grilling, or roasting. Steer clear of all items made from soybeans.

- **Heart-Healthy Fish, such as Salmon, Herring, and Tuna:** Omega-3 fatty acids, which are beneficial to the heart, are abundant in these kinds of seafood. Purchase only "Safe Catch" tuna or other brands that have undergone testing and proven to be mercury-free. Verify that the fish does not come from a fish farm. Many firms market their products as "Wild," yet in reality, they are raised on farms.

- **Nuts, Seeds, and Legumes: 4 to 5 Servings a Week:** Foods in this family, such as almonds, sunflower seeds, kidney beans, peas, lentils, and others, are excellent providers of magnesium, potassium, and protein. Because nuts are higher in calories, omega-6 oils, and glutamate, you should be mindful of how much and how often you eat them. One serving is made up of things like 1/3 cup of nuts, 2 tablespoons of nut butter or seeds, or 1/2 cup of cooked beans or peas.

- **Fats and Oils: 2 to 3 Servings a Day:** The DASH diet places an emphasis on the healthful monounsaturated fats and aims to achieve a balanced diet by keeping total fat to less than 30% of daily calories. This has been shown false. The fats with omega-6 are the most dangerous. As long as one consumes fewer carbohydrates, they can ingest more fat—up to 30%.

The Countless Mediterranean Diet

Based on the food habits of people in 1960s Greece and Italy, research confirm the health advantages of the Mediterranean diet. In addition to having the lowest rates of chronic illnesses like cancer and heart disease, the locals also follow a dietary pattern that is great for liver health, according to recent studies. The Mediterranean diet excludes foods like deli meats, hot dogs, sausages, cookies, cakes, pies, brownies, ice cream, and other desserts, as well as sugary drinks, from the diet. A person on a Mediterranean diet also avoids refined oils (canola, soy, and cottonseed) and processed foods that contain them, as well as processed trans fats like margarine. Olive oil is the main source of fat for them. People who follow the Mediterranean diet base their diets on the following foods:

- **Vegetables:** Broccoli, kale, spinach, onions, cauliflower, carrots, Brussels sprouts, cucumbers, etc.
- **Fruits:** a variety of fruits and vegetables, such as melons, figs, oranges, pears, blueberries, raspberries, blackberries, apples, bananas, and grapes. Due to their high fructose content, they should only be consumed in moderation. Sugar-free fruit powders are the best.

- **Nuts and seeds:** Nuts like walnuts, hazelnuts, cashews, macadamia nuts, sunflower seeds, pumpkin seeds, etc. Once again, some have excessive glutamate and omega-6 oil content.

- **Legumes:** legumes, chickpeas, peanuts, peas, beans, etc. Since all are strong in lectins, they must be thoroughly cooked.

- **Tubers:** potatoes, turnips, yams, sweet potatoes, etc. The high glycemic index list includes Irish potatoes.

- **Whole grains:** Pasta, whole wheat, whole-grain bread, rye, barley, corn, buckwheat, and whole-oats. Once more, these have significant levels of lectins, glutamate, and gluten.

- **Fish and seafood:** seafood such as shrimp, oysters, clams, crab, mussels, sardines, trout, tuna, and mackerel. Consume only seafood low or free of mercury.

- **Poultry:** Chicken, duck, turkey, etc. Only organically raised.

- **Eggs:** Chicken, quail, duck eggs. (Organic)

- **Dairy.** Cheese, yogurt, Greek yogurt, etc. Avoid all of these.

- **Herbs and spices:** Garlic, basil, mint, rosemary, sage, nutmeg, cinnamon, pepper, etc.
- **Healthy fats:** Extra virgin olive oil, olives, avocados, and olive oil.
- **Beverages:** Water is advised as the primary hydration option. One glass of red wine each day is considered a modest amount. This is optional, and anyone suffering from alcoholism or liver impairment should stay away from it. Coffee and white or green tea are fine, but stay away from fruit juices and drinks with added sugar. Monk fruit juice is the only artificial sweetener you should use.

Consuming No Gluten May Help Your Liver

Some people, especially those with celiac disease and gluten sensitivity, may find it difficult to digest gluten, which is a combination of two proteins that is most frequently found in wheat.

Consuming gluten-free food is essential if you have celiac disease. However, it's also better if you've discovered that you have a sensitivity to gluten-containing meals. Everyone is harmed by too much gluten—not only those who identify as "gluten sensitive." Gluten is added to modern processed foods in excess of what is naturally present. Seeking out these naturally gluten-free food groups is the most economical and healthful method to adhere to the gluten-free diet. These food groups include:

- Fruits
- Vegetables
- Meat and poultry
- Fish
- Beans, legumes, and nuts

Although the seeds of pure wheatgrass and barley grass contain gluten, improper harvesting or processing can contaminate the plant. Grain items containing gluten are not allowed in gluten-free diets, but rice, millet, quinoa, and buckwheat are still acceptable. GMO-free veggies like cauliflower and zucchini, as well as corn and quinoa, are used to make gluten-free pastas. Moreover, items including salad dressings, soup, French fries, energy bars, and soy sauce contain gluten. Even if a food is labeled as "gluten-free," it is still important to study the contents because food producers are not compelled to include allergies on labels. On its website (www.celiac.org), the Celiac Disease Foundation provides details on ingredient lists, meal plans, and food lists.